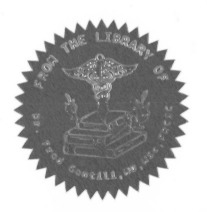

SEMINARS IN NEUROLOGICAL SURGERY SERIES

Vascular Malformations and Fistulas of the Brain

Sponsored by the
Subcommittee on Continuing Education II
(Expanded Program),
American Association of Neurological Surgeons,
and Congress of Neurological Surgeons

Editors

Robert R. Smith, M.D.
Professor and Chairman
Department of Neurosurgery
University of Mississippi
Medical Center
Jackson, Mississippi

Armin F. Haerer, M.D.
Professor of Neurology
University of Mississippi
Medical Center
Jackson, Mississippi

William F. Russell, M.D.
Assistant Professor of Radiology
University of Mississippi
Medical Center
Jackson, Mississippi

Raven Press ■ New York

Raven Press, 1140 Avenue of the Americas, New York, New York 10036

Made in the United States of America

Library of Congress Cataloging in Publication Data
Main entry under title:

Vascular malformations and fistulas of the brain.
  (Seminars in neurological surgery series)
  Includes bibliographical references and indexes.
  1. Brain—Blood-vessels—Abnormalities. 2. Fistula,
Arteriovenous—Surgery. 3. Brain—Blood-vessels—Surgery.
I. Smith, Robert Ray. II. Haerer, Armin F. III. Russell,
William F. (William Frazier), 1942-   . IV. Committee
on Continuing Education in Neurosurgery. Subcommittee on
Continuing Education II (Expanded Program) V. Series.
RD594.2.V37   616.8′1   81-40371
ISBN 0-89004-683-2

Preface

During recent years, advances in diagnostic and therapeutic armamentaria have led to a conceptual renaissance relating to vascular malformations and fistulas of the brain. This volume was developed in the belief that technological achievements, exciting as they are, should not proceed without due regard for traditional views and must be built upon a firm understanding of the natural history of the lesion. Although modern technical advances may have widespread application, the clinical material is embodied in small case series and has never received careful scrutiny, especially that which comes across interdisciplinary lines.

This book is the outgrowth of a seminar which afforded the opportunity for free interchange among radiologists, neurosurgeons, neurologists, pathologists, and ophthalmologists. A bibliography has also been included at the end of each chapter for the reader who desires further reference. Because many of the mechanical advancements have not been described in print, each author has been encouraged to elaborate on these techniques, to be free and open in his discussion of complications and above all, to keep all instructions simple and straightforward.

The book should find an audience among all of those interested in vascular malformations and among all those who manage patients who harbor these rather rare lesions.

The Editors

Acknowledgments

The editors are grateful to the many distinguished contributors to this volume. We express special gratitude to Wally Conerly of Continuing Medical Education at the University of Mississippi Medical Center and to his staff. To Dee Clinton for preparing and watching over the manuscripts, we owe appreciation. To Melanie McClain, Sarah Plagge, Betty Rosenbaum, and Dewanna Crawford, we are thankful for secretarial assistance. To Raven Press, without whose help this volume would not have been possible, we offer thanks for assistance in organizing the seminar and arranging for its publication. We would also like to acknowledge the assistance of the joint committees of the American Association of Neurological Surgeons and the Congress of Neurological Surgeons.

Contents

Contributors

Marshall B. Allen, Jr., M.D.
Department of Neurosurgery
The Medical College of Georgia
Augusta, Georgia 30912

Jose Bebin, M.D.
Department of Pathology
University of Mississippi Medical Center
Jackson, Mississippi 39216

Wayne D. Beveridge, M.D.
Department of Neurosurgery
The Medical College of Georgia
Augusta, Georgia 30912

Betty Brooks, M.D.
Department of Radiology
The Medical College of Georgia
Augusta, Georgia 30912

Larry V. Carson, M.D.
Department of Neurosurgery
The Medical College of Georgia
Augusta, Georgia 30912

Gerard Debrun, M.D.
Department of Neurosurgery
University Hospital
London, Ontario Canada N6A 5A5

Frank M. Eggers, M.D.
Department of Neuroradiology
Cincinnati General Hospital
Cincinnati, Ohio 45267

W. M. Flowers, M.D.
Department of Radiology
University of Mississippi Medical Center
Jackson, Mississippi 39116

Eugene D. George, COL M.D.
Department of Neurosurgery
Walter Reed Army Medical Center
Washington, D. C. 20012

Armin F. Haerer, M.D.
Department of Neurology
University of Mississippi Medical Center
Jackson, Mississippi 39216

P. S. Holla, M.D.
Department of Neurosurgery
University of Mississippi Medical Center
Jackson, Mississippi 39216

Robert R. Lukin, M.D.
Department of Radiology
Cincinnati General Hospital
Cincinnati, Ohio 45267

Clinton E. Massey, M.D.
Department of Neurosurgery
The Medical College of Georgia
Augusta, Georgia 30912

James McLennan, M.D.
Department of Neurosurgery
Cincinnati General Hospital
Cincinnati, Ohio 45267

Chikayuki Ochiai, M.D.
Department of Neurosurgery
University of Tokyo
Tokyo, Japan 7-2-1

Larry Parker, M.D.
Department of Neuro-Ophthalmology
University of Mississippi Medical Center
Jackson, Mississippi 39216

Dwight Parkinson, M.D.
Department of Neurosurgery
University of Manitoba
Winnipeg, Manitoba Canada R3E 0W3

F. L. M. Peeters, M.D.
Department of Diagnostic Radiology
University of Amsterdam
The Netherlands

Paul H. Pevsner, M.D.
Department of Neuroradiology
Walter Reed Army Medical Center
Washington, D. C. 20012

W. F. Russell, M.D.
Department of Radiology
University of Mississippi Medical Center
Jackson, Mississippi 39216

Isamu Saito, M.D.
Department of Neurosurgery
University of Tokyo
Tokyo, Japan 7-2-1

Keiji Sano, M. D.
Department of Neurosurgery
University of Tokyo
Tokyo, Japan 7-2-1

Edward E. Smith, M.D.
Department of Pathology
University of Mississippi Medical Center
Jackson, Mississippi 39216

Robert R. Smith, M.D.
Department of Neurosurgery
University of Mississippi Medical Center
Jackson, Mississippi 39216

John M. Tew, Jr., M.D.
Department of Neurosurgery
Good Samaritan Hospital
Cincinnati, Ohio 45220

Thomas A. Tomsick, M.D.
Department of Radiology
Cincinnati General Hospital
Cincinnati, Ohio 45267

A. J. M. van der Werf, M.D.
Department of Neurosurgery
University of Amsterdam
The Netherlands

F. Yaghmai, M.D.
Department of Pathology
The Medical College of Georgia
Augusta, Georgia 30912

Vascular Malformations, edited by
R. R. Smith, A. Haerer and W. F. Russell.
Raven Press, New York © 1982.

Arteriovenous Malformations of the Brain: Some Comments on their Natural History

Armin F. Haerer

*University of Mississippi Medical Center, Department of Neurology,
Jackson, Mississippi 39216*

Arteriovenous malformations (AVMs) of the brain have been recognized since the middle of the last century (1,5). Several authors have recently described the natural history of these lesions, based on series of variable sizes and follow-ups (1–5).

The present communication presents a current series of AVMs from a southern medical center and attempts to define further some of the features of the natural history of these lesions. Special attention has been placed on the size of the malformations and on their occurrence in different population groups. The literature contains little information concerning differences in occurrence of AVMs of the brain among the various races, especially between whites and blacks in the United States.

Arteriovenous malformations are said to comprise between 1.5 and 4% of verified intracranial masses (5). According to some authors (1,2), they are more common in males than in females, but other authors find less of a difference (3). These lesions are said to be congenital, arising at an early fetal stage (about 3 weeks) when there is division into primitive arteries, capillaries, and veins (6). There is thought to be an arrest in development which results in the formation of direct arteriolar to venous communications without an intervening capillary bed. Presumably, the malformation is transformed and acquires additional arterial contributions during development, and eventually, therefore, results in the occurrence of symptoms later in life. Arteriovenous malformations are said to occur about one-tenth as often as intracranial aneurysms, and only some 2,000 new cases are reported in the United States each year (6).

Much disagreement is found in the literature concerning the recommended treatment for AVMs. The subject is far too complex to be covered in a short review. The interested reader is referred to the more comprehensive studies that address the subject (1–3,5,7,9). A fairly large recent series is that reported by Morello and Borghi (2). It includes a lengthy discussion of successes with surgical versus non-surgical treatments carried out by many different authors. That discussion concludes that the only useful surgical method for dealing with angiomas of the brain is removal, since in most cases the risk of operative mortality is much less than that of hemorrhage. The authors mention that with conservative treatment 20% of the patients will die from a hemorrhage, whereas only one-tenth will die after radical excision. It will be shown that the mortality in the present series is less for both operative and conservative treatments. The definitions used for operable and inoperable AVMs and the skill of the individual surgeon surely must influence the prognosis.

For lesions that are not surgically totally removable there exists a great division of opinion as to the most prudent course to follow. Conservative supportive therapy, shunting procedures for hydrocephalus if necessary, treatment of seizures and headaches, embolization of the lesion, irradiation, trapping or partial ligation of feeders are all methods that are advocated for the control of the more difficult-to-manage AVMs of the brain. Newer approaches are being tried and are being reported periodically in current literature.

Similarly, there is considerable variation in the literature concerning the frequency with which AVMs tend to bleed. The obvious explanation for the variability in the literature is that different centers have different referral patterns and some are more aggressive in studying their patients than others. The opinions concerning the likelihood of AVMs to rebleed once they have bled are less divergent, on the other hand.

The location of the lesions and the feeding vessels that contribute to the makeup of an AVM vary somewhat in their frequency from center to center and are probably due more to differences in definition than true occurrences.

METHODS

All medical records of patients diagnosed as having AVMs of the brain from 1965 to 1978 at the University of Mississippi Medical Center and the Veterans Administration Center in Jackson were reviewed. The patient data were abstracted from the records and an effort was made to obtain follow-up on everyone of the patients so diagnosed. Follow-ups were made by chart review, by personal examination of patients, by follow-up letters, and by telephone calls.

RESULTS

A total number of 81 patients with AVMs of the brain was found. Table 1 summarizes the general patient data. There were 52 males of whom 12 were Veterans Hospital patients; thus at the University Medical Center there were 40 males and

TABLE 1. *General patient data*

Total number of patients	81
Males	52 (includes 12 from Veterans Hospital)
Females	29
Blacks	34
Whites	47

All patients were symptomatic from the AVMs.

TABLE 2. *Ages of onset*

Age of onset of first symptoms[a]
    Range 0–64 years
    Average 26.0 years

Average age of onset of symptoms by race and sex
    White males: 24 years
    White females: 26 years
    Black males: 28 years
    Black females: 24 years

[a]Excludes 2 patients with vein of Galen aneurysms.

29 females. The overall distribution of 34 blacks and 47 whites roughly conforms to the racial distribution in the State of Mississippi. All patients were symptomatic from the AVMs.

Table 2 details the ages of onset of symptoms. No obvious differences are apparent between whites and blacks, or males and females. The median age of onset was 26 years with a very wide range from 0 to 64 years.

Presenting symptoms are shown in Table 3. Headache was most common, followed by loss of consciousness and seizures of generalized or focal nature, and less frequently by other neurologic disturbances.

Presenting signs most commonly were (Table 4) focal neurologic disturbances; bruits were present in the head in 16% and in the neck in 7%.

Two-thirds of the patients were at rest or in light physical activity during the onset of their subarachnoid bleeding (Table 5).

A family history of a similar disorder was found in 3 of 81 patients (Table 6).

Associated disorders (Table 7) occurred infrequently among the 81 patients with AVMs. Heart murmur occurred in 6 patients, hypertension was surprisingly infrequent. Aneurysms were present in 3 patients in addition to their AVMs. Polycy-

TABLE 3. *Presenting symptoms in 81 patients*[a]

Symptom	% of patients
Headache	72%
Altered consciousness	35%
Seizures, grand mal	33%
Seizures, focal	26%
Focal weakness	10%
Diplopia	6%
Tinnitus	4%
Backache	3%
Ataxia	2%
Vertigo	1%
Sensory disturbances	1%

[a]Nausea/vomiting excluded.

TABLE 4. *Presenting signs in 81 patients*

Presenting sign	% of patients
Paresis or paralysis	53%
Nuchal rigidity	28%
Bruits of head	16%
Aphasia	11%
Third-nerve palsy	11%
Bruits in neck	7%
Hemianopsia	7%
Nystagmus	5%
Facial palsy without body weakness	4%
Others:	1–3% each
Dysarthria	
Cerebellar signs	
Sensory loss	
Brain syndrome, etc.	

TABLE 5. *Physical activity at time of onset of bleed, if known*

Strenuous	34%
Light	66%

TABLE 6. *Family history of AVMs[a]*

2 had multiple relatives
1 had a single relative

[a]3 out of 81 patients.

TABLE 7. *Associated disorders among 81 patients*

Disorder	No. of patients
Heart murmur	6
Significant hypertension	5
Ulcers, duodenal	4
Congestive heart failure	3
Cerebral aneurysm	3
Glioma	1
Unrelated stroke	2
Polycythemia (>17)	2
AVM of lung	1
Telangiectasias of body	2
Congenital anomalies	2
Hydrocephalus	2

themia was surprisingly uncommon, being reported in only 2 patients. One patient had AVMs elsewhere in his body as well.

Of these studies done, 100% of the angiograms and CAT scans were abnormal in patients with AVMs (Table 8). Lumbar puncture was slightly less sensitive, as were nuclide scans. Skull X-rays were abnormal in only one-third.

TABLE 8. *Abnormal studies in 81 patients*

Study	% abnormal, if done
Skull X-rays	32%
Nuclide scans	76%
Lumbar puncture	79%
CAT scans	100%
Angiograms	100%

TABLE 9. *Location of lesions in 81 patients*

Lesion	No. of patients
Frontal	12
Parietal	19
Temporal	8
Occipital	5
Hemispheric, unilateral	21
Posterior fossa	11
Deep, midline, or bilateral	3
Vein of Galen	2

TABLE 10. *Size of lesion in 81 patients*

Large	49%
Medium	17%
Small	31%
Uncertain	3%

The location of the lesions is summarized in Table 9. The most common locations were in the parietal lobe and unilateral involving the entire hemisphere.

The lesions were preponderantly large (Table 10); only a small number were considered to be medium in size and about one-third were small in size. Lesions exceeding 5 cm in diameter were considered to be large, those 2 to 5 cm were medium, and those less than 2 cm small.

Table 11 lists the feeding vessels of the malformations. Of course, multiple feeding vessels were very common, but the single most common feeding vessel

TABLE 11. *Major feeding vessels in 81 patients*

Vessel	% of patients
Middle cerebral artery	38%
Multiple vessels, unilateral	17%
Multiple vessels, bilateral	12%
Anterior cerebral artery	10%
Basilar-vertebral arery	10%
Posterior cerebral artery	7%
Uncertain	4%

was, as expected, the middle cerebral artery. The external vessels were not included in this compilation of feeding vessels but are, of course, known to be contributors in some patients as well.

As for management (Table 12), the conservative approach was slightly more common than excision; ligation was much less common, and embolization was only done on 4 patients in this series.

TABLE 12. *Treatment of 81 patients[a]*

Treatment	No. of patients
Conservative (includes CSF shunts)	38
Excision of AVM	30
Ligation of feeders	9
Embolization of AVM	4

[a]There were no significant differences in treatment compared to patients' race or sex.

TABLE 13. *Duration of symptoms to time of surgical treatment[a]*

Range: < 1 to 34 years   Average: 5.3 years

[a]Nine patients had symptoms for over 10 years prior to operation.

The duration of symptoms (Table 13) to the time of surgical treatment averaged 5.3 years, with 9 patients having symptoms for over 10 years prior to operation. The range of symptoms prior to surgical treatment was from days to 34 years, emphasizing the unpredictability of these lesions.

Table 14 summarizes data for the onset of the first bleed. Fifty-eight percent of all patients in this series bled; the average age of the first bleed was 28 years. There was no significant difference between races and sexes in the time of onset of these bleeds.

TABLE 14. *Age of onset of first bleed*

Of 81 patients, 47 bled (58% of all patients)
Onset of first bleed ranged from 1 to 64 years.
Average age of onset: 28 years.

Age of onset (average) of first bleed compared to
patient's race or sex:
White males: 23 years
White females: 26 years
Black males: 34 years
Black females: 27 years

The relationship of the initial symptoms to the first bleed is of some interest and is summarized in Table 15. Of 47 patients who bled, only 4 did not have the bleeding episode as their first symptom. Thus, the bleeding episode is the first symptom in the overwhelming majority of those patients with AVMs who are going to bleed.

TABLE 15. *Relationship of initial symptoms to first bleed*

Of 47 patients who bled, only 4 did *not* have the bleeding episode as their first symptom. The duration of
their symptoms was 2–22 (average 8) years, prior
to the bleed in those 4 patients.

TABLE 16. *Treatment related to size of lesion*

Patients with small lesions
Treated conservatively   36%
Excision   56%
Ligation   8%

Patients with medium-sized lesions
Treated conservatively   31%
Excision   69%

Patients with large lesions
Treated conservatively   65%
Excision   10%
Ligation   15%
Embolization   10%

Treatment is related to size of the lesions in Table 16 as determined in this retrospective analysis. The percentage of patients treated conservatively is higher among those with large (and thus surgically difficult) lesions.

Rebleeds occurred in 16% of all patients, or 28% of all those who bled (Table 17). The timing of rebleeds occurred on the average 6 years after the initial one, but the range extended from less than 1 to 32 years after the first bleed.

TABLE 17. *Data on rebleeds*

1. Initial bleed occurred in 47 of 81 patients (58%).
   Second bleed occurred in 16% of all patients, or
      28% of those who bled.
   Third bleed occurred in 4% of all, or 6% of those
      that bled.
   Fourth, fifth and sixth bleed occurred only in one
      patient (1% of all), or 2% of those that bled.

2. Timing of rebleeds.
   Range: < 1 to 32 years (after first bleed)
   Average: 6 years
   Of 13 patients who had rebleeds, 10 did so in less
      than 5 years from first episode.

The overall mortality was 16% (Table 18). 3.7% died during the initial hospi-talization, but only 2 patients died from the initial bleeds. Of the 10 patients who died after discharge, only 6 died from rebleeds; thus only 8 patients, or somewhat less than 10%, died during the entire follow-up period from bleeds or rebleeds. There was no significant racial nor sex preponderance in the mortality figures.

Table 19 notes that over 95% of the patients could be followed up. The average follow-up was 7 years with a range of 0 to 38 years. Again, there are no marked differences in the duration of follow-up by race or sex.

Tables 20, 21, and 22 deal with outcome during follow-up and outcome by treatment and by size of the lesion. About 40% of the patients remained the same and 40% were better during the overall follow-up; worse conditions were described in 4%, and 16% died. The outcome of conservative treatment was not as good as that of excision, whereas such small numbers of patients had embolization or ligation that no significant conclusions can be drawn about these forms of treatment.

TABLE 18. *Analysis of deaths among 81 patients*

1. Total deaths during follow-up period were 13 patients or 16%.

2. Of those, 3 (3.7%) died during initial hospitalization,
      2 from bleeds, 1 from cardiac causes.

3. 10 patients died after discharge.
   Of these, causes of death were:
Rebleed	6 patients
Glioma	1 patient
Leukemia	1 patient
Gangrene	1 patient
Unknown cause	1 patient

4. Of the patients that died there were:
   7 males
   6 females
   7 whites
   6 blacks

TABLE 19. *Data on follow-up of 81 patients*

1. Total number of patients followed is 77/81
   or 95.2%

2. Average duration of follow-up was 7 years,
   range 0–38 years

3. Average duration of follow-up by race and sex
   White males   6.7 years
   White females 7.5 years
   Black males   5.9 years
   Black females 7.4 years

TABLE 20. *Outcome during follow-up of
81 patients, overall*

Better	40%
Same	40%
Worse	4%
Died	16%

TABLE 21. *Outcome by treatment during 7-year follow-up of 81 patients*

Treatment	Outcome			
	% Better	% Same	% Worse	% Died
Conservative treatment	29	42	3	26
Excision	63	37	0	0
Ligation	0	67	11	22
Embolization	50	0	25	25

TABLE 22. *Outcome by size of lesion during 7-year
follow-up of 81 patients*

Size	Outcome			
	% Better	% Same	% Worse	% Dead
Small lesions	64	36	0	0
Medium	36	64	0	0
Large	23	37	8	32

However, the outcome during the 7-year follow-up of these patients was significantly related to the size of the lesion, there being no mortality at all in patients with small or medium-sized lesions and about one-third mortality in those with large lesions. Improvement in those with medium-sized lesions, however, was not as frequent as in those with small lesions. This result tends to confirm the desirability of a radical excision of AVMs if they are small or medium sized. Mortality in this series did not seem to be related to the site of the lesion (Table 23).

TABLE 23. *Mortality among 81 patients related to site of lesion (total dead, 13) during average 7-year follow-up*

Site of lesion	No. of patients
Frontal	1
Temporal	1
Parietal	4
Posterior fossa	2
Unilateral hemispheric	2[a]
Bilateral hemispheric	1
Deep	2[b]

[a]One died in hospital.
[b]Both died in hospital.

DISCUSSION

In terms of the approximate population base at this center, the number of AVMs that are diagnosed corresponds approximately to the expected number, if some 2,000 new cases are said to occur in the United States annually (6). Furthermore, there is no obviously detectable difference in the occurrence and in the natural history of the AVMs of the brain between whites and blacks in the present series, insofar as the patients represent a cross-section of the population of this area.

The first symptoms of AVMs in many reported series occurred during the second and third decades of life, in agreement with the present series. Malformations have been described as equally common in the right and left hemispheres and are most frequent in the parietal region. The present series is similar. The cooperative aneurysm study (5), which reported 545 cases of AVMs, describes the most common symptoms as convulsions, hemorrhage, headaches, progressive neurological deficit, and mental deterioration. Considering the differences in listing of signs and symptoms, there is little disagreement between the present series and the cooperative aneurysm study. The ratio of male to female patients in the cooperative aneurysm study was 1.1 to 1, slightly lower than in the present series where 40 males were included with 29 females at the University Medical Center, excluding the male patients from the Veterans Hospital facility. Forty-four percent of AVMs of the brain were diagnosed in patients between the ages of 21 and 40 years, again similar to the present series.

The recurrence of hemorrhages in AVMs was described as 6% by Tönnis and colleagues (8). The cooperative aneurysm study (5), on the other hand, states that for supratentorial malformations the rebleeding rate was 23%. In the present series it was 28%. The differences are probably due to differences in the type and duration of follow-ups, the present series having a rather lengthy and fairly complete follow-up. The mortality rate due to hemorrhage in patients with bleeding AVMs in the cooperative study was described as 10%, this being significantly higher than in the present series. Again, differences between series of patients, no doubt, are due to differences in referral patterns. The rapidity of referral to a center may influence the mortality rate. Also, the operative mortality in the cooperative study was 14% for AVMs, higher than in the present series. The decision to operate may have been influenced by the likelihood of having a low mortality in the present series.

It is said that only 6% of AVMs are located in the posterior fossa (6). The somewhat higher incidence of posterior fossa malformations in the present series is probably related to more adequate study in recent years with CAT scans and more complete angiography, revealing more of the small posterior fossa malformations.

There has always been a question as to what happens to the size of AVMs. The present series has no good data about their change in size with time. However, the series of Stein and Wolpert (6) mentions that in 9 cases that were followed angiographically for many years, a third of the lesions enlarged, a third remained unchanged, and a third actually became smaller. Further work is clearly needed to clarify what happens to the size of AVMs that are not specifically treated surgically.

In a number of studies, hemorrhage occurred in about 50% of AVMs, but in children it may be the initial sign in as many as 85% of patients (6). The present study has only a few individuals in the childhood age and cannot comment on this difference. Stein and Wolpert (6) mention that in a recent series 27 of 41 angiomas were diagnosed by CAT scan, and this is not surprising, since the accuracy of the CAT scan is still improving. In the present series all patients that had a CAT scan and eventually were diagnosed as having an AVM had an abnormality on the CAT scan.

Perrett (4) notes that there seems to be little variability from slight to severe physical activity during the occurrence of bleeds from cerebral AVMs. That certainly seems to be confirmed in the present series in which about two-thirds of the bleeds began during periods of relative inactivity.

Perret (4) reports an overall mortality of 11% from hemorrhage from AVMs. In the present series, 8 of 81 or just under 10% died of hemorrhage initially or during the prolonged follow-up period. Perret also states that the size of the lesion is not related to the presenting symptoms, the prognosis following hemorrhage does not correlate with the location of the lesion nor the age of the patient. These statements are confirmed by the present series, although detailed data are not presented.

CONCLUSIONS

A 7-year average follow-up of all diagnosed AVMs of the brain at this medical center finds no significant difference in the occurrence or outcome between whites and blacks. The mortality is less than in many reported series. The outcome is best with complete surgical excision and is improved in patients with small as compared to large lesions.

REFERENCES

1. Forster, D. M. C., Steiner, L., and Hakanson, S. (1972): Arteriovenous malformations of the brain. A long-term clinical study. *J. Neurosurg.*, 37:562–570.
2. Morello, G., and Borghi, G. P. (1973): Cerebral angiomas. A report of 154 personal cases and a comparison between the results of surgical excision and conservative management. *Acta Neurochir.*, 28:135–155.
3. Perret, G. (1975): The epidemiology and clinical course of arteriovenous malformations. In: *Cerebral Angiomas: Advances in Diagnosis and Therapy*, edited by H. W. Pia, J. R. W. Gleave, E. Grote, and J. Zierski, pp. 21–26. Springer Pub. Co., New York.
4. Perret, G. (1975): Conservative management of inoperable arteriovenous malformations. In: *Cerebral Angiomas: Advances in Diagnosis and Therapy*, edited by H. W. Pia, J. R. W. Gleave, E. Grote, and J. Zierski, pp. 268–270. Springer Pub. Co., New York.
5. Perret, G., and Nishioka, H. (1969): Arteriovenous maliformations. In: *Intracranial Aneurysms and Subarachnoid Hemorrhage, A Cooperative Study*, edited by A. L. Sahs, G. E. Perret, H. B. Locksley, and H. Nishioka, Chapter 12, pp. 200–222. Springer Pub. Co., Philadelphia.
6. Stein, B. M., and Wolpert, S. M. (1980): Arteriovenous malformations of the brain. I. Current concepts and treatment. *Arch. Neurol.*, 37:1–5.
7. Stein, B. M., and Wolpert, S. M. (1980): Arteriovenous malformations of the brain. II. Current concepts and treatment. *Arch. Neurol.*, 37:69–75.
8. Tonnis, W., Schiefer, W., and Walter, W. (1958): Signs and symptoms of supratentorial arteriovenous aneurysms. *J. Neurosurg.*, 15:471–480.
9. Walter, W. (1975): Conservative treatment of cerebral arteriovenous angiomas. In: *Cerebral Angiomas: Advances in Diagnosis and Therapy*, edited by H. W. Pia, J. R. W. Gleave, E. Grote, and J. Zierski, pp. 271–273.Spinger Pub. Co., New York.

Vascular Malformations, edited by
R. R. Smith, A. Haerer and W. F. Russell.
Raven Press, New York © 1982.

Vascular Malformations of the Brain

Jose Bebin and Edward E. Smith

*Department of Pathology, University of Mississippi Medical Center,
Jackson, Mississippi 39216*

Malformations of the cerebral blood vessels are far from rare, and the problems they produce frequently are a challenge to the neurosurgeon and neurologist. Although some of these lesions have been regarded as neoplasms (angiomas), the prevalent opinion is that most are not true neoplasms but are probably congenital malformations of the blood vessels resulting from a defect in angiogenesis. The occasional association of vascular anomalies of the brain with those of skin, bone, and meninges can best be explained by a maldevelopment occurring early in life. Despite this, they are usually asymptomatic until adulthood—typically in the second through the fifth decades—when they may then produce seizures, hemorrhage, or symptoms of a space-occupying lesion.

Whatever the origin of the anomalies, some authors believe that vascular malformations may eventually acquire a true neoplastic character and that the symptoms they elicit may be the result of regressive changes in the adjacent brain tissue as a consequence of repeated hemorrhages and secondary gliosis. The development of arteriovenous communications in these lesions can also lead to progressive enlargement of the lesions and increasing symptomatology.

The classification of the vascular malformations of the brain has been the subject of considerable discussion, and the extensive literature on this topic reflects a varying and, at times, confusing nomenclature. The type of vessel constituting a malformation has led to the designations of arterial angiomas, venous angiomas, capillary angiomas, and telangiectasias. The difficulties involved in the identification of vessel type has produced terms such as varix arteriale and varix aneurysmatic. Emphasis on the congenital origin has given us the terms vascular hamartoma and congenital angioma. "Arteriovenous malformation" (AVM) or "arteriovenous aneurysm" are now more popular than the term arteriovenous angioma.

The classical reviews on the pathology of vascular malformations of the brain are those of Cushing and Bailey (9); Bergstrand et al. (3); van Bogaert (30); Noran (20), and more recently, Russell and Rubinstein (24) and McCormick (16).

As noted, most authors accept that these lesions are developmental malformations of the blood vessels and are not true neoplasms. Russell and Rubinstein (24), among others, have considered them to be a variety of hamartoma of Albrecht, but this term has not received wide acceptance. Bergstrand (4) regarded any attempts to classify the lesions as either neoplasms or as malformations to be misleading, since he believed that the two concepts are not mutually exclusive. For example, this author considered hemangioblastomas to be vascular malformations that have acquired an autonomous growth.

13

In the earliest classification by Virchow (31), vascular malformations were divided into two groups: cavernous angiomas and racemose angiomas. The outstanding characteristic of the first group was that vascular walls in the lesions were common to more than one vascular lumen and that no parenchymatous tissue intervened between the vessels. In the second group, the lesions consisted of aggregates of individual vessels separated by parenchymatous tissue. The latter group was further subdivided according to the character of the vessels into (a) telangiectasia (angioma with capillary-like vessels), (b) *angioma racemosum venosum* (angioma with venous type vessels), (c) *angioma racemosum arteriale* (angioma of arteries),and (d) *aneurysm arteriale et venosum* (AVM where blood flows directly from artery to vein without an interposed capillary bed). To this classification Bergstrand (4) added two new groups: the *angioreticuloma* (angioblastoma) of the cerebellum and medulla oblongata, and the *angioglioma* (of Roussy and Oberling), which is a combination of glial and vascular elements.

Bergstrand's Classification
 1. Angioma cavernosum
 2. Angioma racemosum
    a. Telangiectasia
    b. Sturge–Weber disease
    c. Angioma racemosum arteriale
    d. Angioma racemosum venosum
    e. Angioma arteriovenosum
 3. Angioreticuloma
 4. Angioglioma

It is debatable whether a telangiectasia should be considered to be a variety of angioma racemosum, and whether the term "angioreticuloma" is preferable to the more widely accepted "hemangioblastoma." The "angioglioma" may very well also be an hemangioblastoma.

A decisive attempt at separation of vascular lesions into malformations and true neoplasms was made by Cushing and Bailey in 1928 (9) with the following classification:

I. Cerebral vascular malformations
    a. Telangiectasia
    b. Venous angioma
    c. Arterial (arteriovenous) angioma
II. Hemangioblastomas

Here the emphasis is placed on the nature of the interstitial tissue of the lesion. Vascular neoplasms (hemangioblastomas) have no neural parenchyma between the tumor elements, whereas vascular malformations have neural tissue between the vessels. The presence of brain parenchyma between the component vessels of a vascular lesion is considered of paramount importance in the recognition of the lesion as an anomaly or malformation rather than a neoplasm. Bergstrand (4), in arguing against this distinction, noted that in some cases of vascular malformations interstitial neural tissue was absent and that the vascular malformations were not static, but grew and produced progressive destruction of the adjacent parenchyma, yet on histological examination showed no evidence of cellular proliferation of the vascular elements which would be a necessary criterion for true neoplasia.

The enlargement of a vascular malformation may result from a progressive dilatation of the affected vessels, perhaps due to changes in intravascular pressures and flows, or in some forms, to the development of arteriovenous communications. Alterations within the vessels such as stasis and thrombosis may add further damage to the neighboring tissue, resulting in enlargement of the lesion.

Russell and Rubinstein (24) consider vascular malformations to be hamartomas of blood vessels—congenital anomalies—which, although not true neoplasms, nevertheless resemble tumors in their clinical behavior and pathological features. These authors proposed the following classification:

I. Blood vessel hamartomas (vascular malformations)
  a. Capillary telangiectasias
  b. Cavernous angiomas
  c. Venous and arteriovenous malformations
II. Hemangioblastomas

The discussion which follows will consider only those lesions which can be regarded as vascular malformations in accordance with the above criteria. Included among these are the following: a) Telangiectasias, b) cavernous angiomas, c) venous angiomas, d) Sturge–Weber disease, e) AVMs (arteriovenous aneurysms).

PATHOGENESIS

The earliest development of the blood vascular system was described in detail by Sabin (25). The embryonic vascular system originates from mesenchymal angioblastic cells which initially form clusters. The future blood vessels appear first as solid cords, then the outer cells flatten to become endothelial cells. The inner cells break down into a plasma-like substance, thus forming fluid-filled channels. Initially, these channels are neither arterial nor venous, but represent the structures from which arteries and veins will derive when the channels become linked to the functioning circulatory system.

Five periods in the development of the blood supply to the brain were defined by Streeter (27). These show the special adaptations of the emerging vessels to changing developmental conditions. These stages occur during the earliest embryonic development.

1. *Formation of the primordial head vascular plexus*. Angioblastic differentiation forms solid masses of cells initially arranged into cord-like structures which gradually assume a plexiform configuration.

2. *Blood vessel formation*. The primordial vascular plexus slowly resolves itself into arteries, veins, and capillaries. This plexus appears first over the more rostral portion of the embryonic brain where it differentiates into afferent, efferent, and capillary components. The capillary component remains closely attached to the brain surface, and the more superficial plexus forms larger vascular channels while maintaining communication with the capillary bed. It is during this period that the primary circulation of the brain develops, consisting principally of the capillary bed closely applied to the embryonic brain and supplied by arterial channels from the aortic arch and drained by venous channels leading to the heart. Thus, the first true circulation of the head is established (approximately 4-mm embryo).

3. *Stratification*. With the early differentiation of supporting structures (e.g., dura mater), which are derived from mesoderm, separation of the primitive vascular system into superficial and deep components occurs. The subsequent development of the membranous skull further separates the dural system from the external vascular system which supplies the integument. Thus a pial, dural, and external circulation is established. According to Streeter (27), this occurs in the 12 to 20-mm embryo.

4. *Rearrangement*. Changes in the arrangements of the vascular channels now occur. Some vascular trunks become obliterated as newer branches develop to replace the earlier pattern. This culminates in the constitution of the circle of Willis. This period begins in about the 18 mm embryo and extends into the fetal period. In this stage, the trigeminal and the hypoglossal arteries undergo involution.

5. *Histological development*. Parallel to structural brain development the final morphological differentiation of the blood vessels proceeds, resulting in the formation of morphologically recognizable arteries, veins, and capillaries. This period extends well beyond birth.

There is considerable overlap of these periods. Disturbance or arrest of vascular development during a particular period will determine the type and the location of the vascular malformation which is ultimately observed. If, for example, normal development fails at a particular site in the second period, the vessels of the resulting malformation may be of an indeterminate type due to their undifferentiated nature at this time. Thus, an aberration in this period would be likely to result in a cavernous angioma-like lesion. Conceivably it could also result in the formation of an AVM because of the absence of a capillary network during this period. A disturbance during the period of stratification might determine whether a vascular malformation is located in the scalp, meninges, or brain. Simultaneous defects of more than one stratum may explain the occasional association of vascular nevi of the scalp or the skin with vascular malformations of the dura mater (i.e., dural varices) as well as with vascular malformations of the pia, or of all three together. Gross anomalies of the cerebral circulation may result from alterations of development during the period of rearrangement.

INCIDENCE AND LOCATIONS

In published reports the incidence of vascular malformations of the brain found at autopsy is rather small. In 30,000 autopsies Courville (6) found only 29 (0.1%); namely, 18 telangiectasias, 5 venous angiomas, 5 venous varices, and 1 anteriovenous angioma. An autopsy series from the Institute of Pathology of Vienna by Jellinger (12) disclosed 20 angiomas of the brain in 5,553 autopsies (0.35%). Of these, there were 6 telangiectasias, 1 cavernous angioma, 1 venous angioma, and 12 AVMs. In the neurosurgical literature the reported incidence of vascular malformations of the brain usually varies from 0.5 to 1%. According to Jellinger (12), at the Neurological Institute of Vienna during 1964–1972 the incidence of intracranial angiomas was 3.5% of all intracranial neoplasms. Olivecrona and Ladenheim (21), at the Neurosurgical Clinic of Serafimerlasarettet of Stockholm during 1923–1955, found 125 arteriovenous aneurysms of the carotid and vertebral systems among 5,000 brain tumors, an incidence of approximately 2%. The findings of the Cooperative Study of intracranial aneurysms and subarachnoid hemorrhage (26) included 453 AVMs, of which 421 (93%) were supratentorial and 32 (7%) were infratentorial. Of the supratentorial AVMs, 329 (72%) occurred in a cerebral hemisphere, and 104 (23%) were in the parietal lobes; 81 (18%) were intraventricular or paraventricular involving midline structures; 11 (2%) were in the brainstem, and 21 (5%) were in the cerebellum. McCormick et al. (18) reported a series of 480 patients with 510 vascular malformations of the brain, of which 164 (32%) occurred in the posterior fossa, and 346 (68%) were in the cerebrum.

The location of an intracranial vascular malformation is of paramount importance when surgical excision of the lesion is contemplated. Surgical strategy depends on the accessibility of the lesion, its size and extent, the source of its blood supply, and the possible morbidity resulting from resection. Table 1, modified from Jellinger (12), summarizes the locations of vascular malformations of the brain as reported by various authors. A breakdown of the locations and types of malformations as reported by McCormick et al. (18) is given in Table 2.

Vascular malformations of the brain have been grouped by Olivecrona and Ladenheim (21) according to their vascular supply: malformations supplied principally by external carotid artery (external circulation), and malformations supplied by the internal carotid artery or the vertebral arteries (internal circulation). In the first group, of 7 cases of external carotid artery AVMs these authors found that 6 were

TABLE 1. *Percentage location of brain angiomas*[a]

	Perrett and Nishioka (22)	Berry et al. (5)	Krayenbühl and Yasargil (14)	McCormick et al. (18)	Jellinger (12)
No. of cases	453	527	186	510 autopsies	117 autopsies 83 biopsies
Location					
Cerebral hemisphere	80%	95%	84.6%	70%	77%
Brainstem	2%		2.6%	13%	16%
Cerebellum	5%	5%	9.6%	17%	7%
Diff/multi	2%		3.2%		
Not given	11%				

[a]From Jellinger (12).

TABLE 2. *Brain angiomas: type and location*[a]

Type	Location			
	Cerebral	Cerebellar	Brainstem	Total
Telangiectasias	22	6	32	60
Cavernous angiomas	59	4	10	80
Varix[a]	2	2	2	6
Venous angiomas	46	20	11	77
A-V malformations	217	52	18	287
Total	346	91	73	510

[a]McCormick et al. (18) define as "varix" a single, or occasionally several dilated veins. In our view these lesions might be included among the venous angiomas.

supplied exclusively by branches of the external carotid artery, while one had a small additional contribution from the internal circulation. In 5 cases of intracerebral AVMs, the predominant or exclusive blood supply was from the external carotid artery. This latter group included lesions located in all lobes of the brain. The location of lesions of the second group supplied by the internal carotid–vertebral arteries are listed in Table 3. This series demonstrates that one-half of all AVMs of the brain were located in the distribution of a middle cerebral artery and are supplied by this vessel or its branches. Less common were the AVMs in the distribution of anterior cerebral artery, whereas the least common were those supplied by the posterior cerebral artery. It was noted that lesions located deep within the brain substance may receive additional contributions from the choroidal arteries and from the vessels of choroid plexus.

TELANGIECTASIAS

Telangiectasias (capillary angiomas) of the brain are relatively common but are often discovered only at postmortem examination. They most frequently occur in the pons or white matter of the cerebral hemispheres, but also may be found in the basal ganglia or in the cerebellum.

TABLE 3. *Vascular supply of AVMs of the brain*[a]

Internal carotid artery		107
Anterior cerebral	24	
Anterior + middle cerebral	10	
Middle cerebral	64	
Middle + posterior cerebral	6	
Posterior cerebral	1	
Posterior cerebral + vertebral	3	
Vertebral artery		6
Total		113

[a]From Olivecrona and Ladenheim (21).

Grossly, telangiectasias appear as poorly defined dark areas of discoloration where close examination will disclose a number of minute congested and distended vessels (Fig. 1A). Microscopically a telangiectasia consists of an aggregate of separate, small, dilated, endothelial-lined, capillary-like spaces surrounded by a few strands of collagen and devoid of muscle and elastic fibers. Relatively normal neural tissue separates the individual vessels (Fig. 1B). Rarely, some slight degree of gliosis is present in this parenchyma.

Telangiectasias may be single or multiple and may be associated with other similar lesions in the skin and elsewhere. They may also occur with cavernous angiomas in the same individual. Large hemorrhages have seldom been reported from these lesions.

Osler–Rendu–Weber Disease

This disease is characterized by multiple telangiectasias of the skin and mucosal surfaces but only exceptionally involves the brain. Examples of CNS involvement have been reported by Courville (7) and Heffner and Solitaire (10).

Ataxia Telangiectasia (Louis–Bar Syndrome)

This condition is characterized by an association of conjunctival and facial telangiectasias with leptomeningeal cerebellar telangiectasias, loss of cerebellar Purkinje cells, and a defect of the immunoglobulin system, which is usually reflected as low IgA and IgE.

The literature reports association of multiple CNS telangiectasias with small cavernous angiomas of the skin and other organs (24).

Unna (29) and Russell (23) have suggested that telangiectasias may be transformed into cavernous angiomas by contraction of the fibrous tissue surrounding the communications of the telangiectasias with the vessels of the general circulation, thereby causing dilatation of the telangiectatic vessels and eventually crowding out the parenchyma. Although examples can be found that appear transitional between a telangiectasia and a cavernous angioma, this relationship appears doubtful. If cavernous angiomas represent a later stage of the development of telangiectasias, the incidence of cavernous angiomas should increase in number with age. This has not been supported by the published data, and cavernous angiomas may occur in children and in newborns.

CAVERNOUS ANGIOMAS

These lesions are generally considered to be rare in the CNS; however, their frequency may have been underestimated. McCormick et al. (18) list 59 cavernous angiomas among 346 cerebral angiomas. Russell and Rubinstein (24) studied 32 cases. Cavernous angiomas, depending on their size and location, may be symptomatic and may be a cause of cerebral hemorrhage, although the hemorrhage is rarely massive.

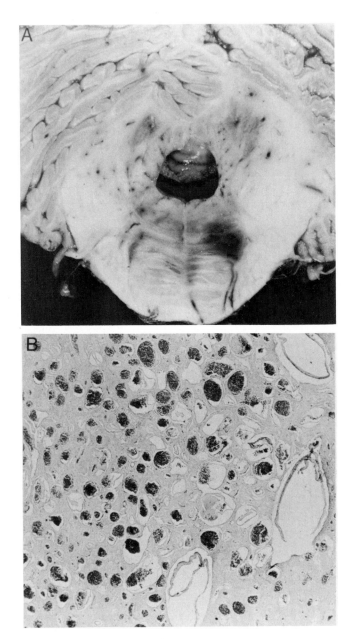

FIG. 1. **A:** A telangiectasia of the pons. **B:** Photomicrograph of this lesion showing multiple dilated capillaries and venules separated by neural tissue (Trichrome, ×17).

Cavernous angiomas generally do not become apparent until adult life. They are more frequent in men than in women. Most are located in the cerebral hemispheres, typically involving the Rolandic region. However, they may be subcortical and may occur in the cerebral white matter or in the basal ganglia. Cavernous angiomas are usually solitary but can be multiple; Russell and Rubinstein (24) mention a case with 42 small cavernous angiomas. The sizes of cavernous angiomas vary greatly. We have studied a cerebral cavernous angioma of the right frontal lobe which measured 5 × 3 × 2 cm (Fig. 2). Most range from a few millimeters to 1 to 2 centimeters in size.

Cavernous angiomas usually are well circumscribed and dark red or hemorrhagic-appearing. They consist of a mass of large irregular vascular spaces distended with blood and separated by fibrous tissue. The adjacent neural tissue may be yellowish or brownish due to previous bleeding. Microscopically they are made up of a multitude of irregularly shaped, endothelial-lined blood channels which are separated by partitions of connective tissue of variable thicknesses. Old and recent hemorrhages, organizing thrombi, hemosiderin pigment, and calcifications may be found in these lesions. Usually no prominent arteries or veins occur in the vicinity of a cavernous angioma.

As noted, cavernous angiomas of the brain may be associated with similar lesions in other organs such as liver, kidneys, or skin. Russell and Rubinstein (24) noted that this association occurs more frequently in cases of multiple CNS cavernous angiomas. The brain of a 48-year-old woman who had multiple small cavernous angiomas in the cerebrum and meninges and also an enormous cavernous angioma of the liver is illustrated in Fig. 3.

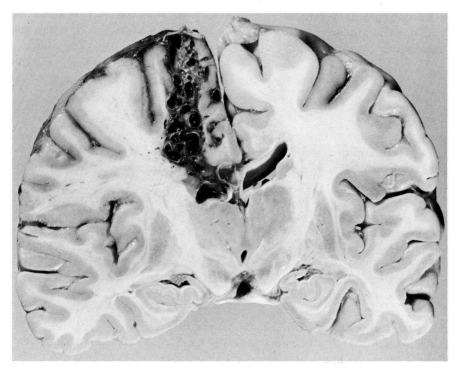

FIG. 2. A large cavernous angioma of the right frontoparietal region.

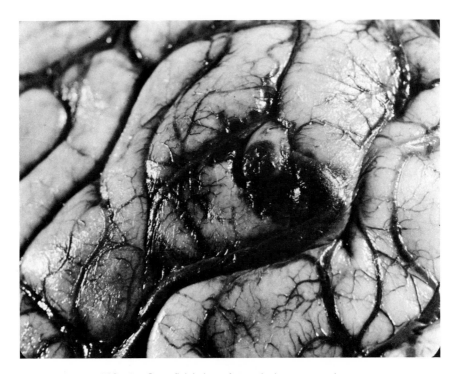

FIG. 4. Superficial view of a cortical venous angioma.

double contours seen in the skull films are due to visualization in depth of opposing surfaces of the widened sulci. Subcortical white matter often shows considerable demyelination.

Although the pathogenesis of Sturge–Weber disease is poorly understood, the association of cutaneous and pial angiomas points to a defect occurring in the embryonic primitive vascular plexus prior to the formation of the separate vasculatures of the skin, skull, and meninges. According to Alexander and Norman, in "the early stages of development the small telencephalic vesicle and the eye are closely approximated and the integument of the embryo's forehead might well share that part of the vascular plexus which supplies the occipital portions of the brain. The later anatomical separation of these two vascular territories occurs as the result of the subsequent growth backwards of the hemisphere" (1). The rarity of dural and cranial angiomas remains unexplained. The origin of the intracranial calcification is also unknown.

ARTERIOVENOUS MALFORMATIONS (ARTERIOVENOUS ANEURYSMS)

These are the most frequent and best known vascular malformations of neurosurgical practice. The literature on this lesion is extensive.

Cerebral AVMs typically consist of complex congeries of vessels of various sizes and wall thicknesses in which both arterial and venous elements occur. Usually

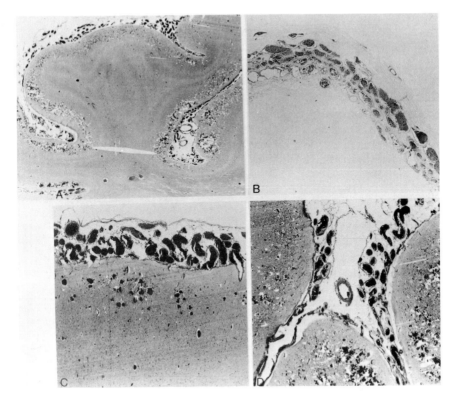

FIG. 5. Sturge–Weber disease. **A:** Occipital cortex showing pial venous angioma and extensive calcifications (H and E, × 2.5); **B:** Venous angioma of choroid from the same case (H and E, × 15; **C** and **D:** Leptomenigeal venous angiomas with calcification in superficial cortical layers (H and E, × 15).

arteriovenous shunts exist between the dilated arterial and venous components of the lesion.

Embryologically, cerebral vessels first develop in the pia mater; hence AVMs are frequently superficial, although some lesions may be concealed from view in the depth of a sulcus. An AVM may extend deeply into the brain in a somewhat wedge-shaped fashion and may even reach and project into a lateral ventricle.

Arteriovenous malformations are most commonly encountered in the territory of a middle cerebral artery, although they may occur anywhere in the cerebral hemispheres including the choroid plexuses. They are less frequent in the brainstem and the cerebellum, and are uncommon in the spinal cord.

Wyburn-Mason (34) reported the rare association of an AVM of the midbrain with vascular anomalies of the retina and optic pathways and a trigeminal cutaneous nevus.

The meninges overlying the tangled vessels of an AVM are often thickened and sometimes brownish-yellow due to previous hemorrhages. Adjacent cerebral convolutions are often atrophic. The cerebral atrophy, the degree of extension of the lesion into the brain, and the striking variation in calibers and thicknesses of the constituent vessels is best appreciated on cross-sections of a resected specimen (Fig. 6). Secondary alterations in the blood vessels often occur. These include fibrosis, antheromatous changes, and calcifications of the vessel walls. Atrophy and gliosis of the adjacent brain tissue is usually present.

At surgery, AVMs may be dramatic and one must agree with Cushing and Bailey (9) that "it is improbable that the postmortem appearance could give more than a faint idea of what the actual pulsating snarl of vessels was during life."

On microscopic examination, some of the vessels of an AVM have characteristics of arteries and others of veins, but most of the vessels show pathological alterations consisting of unequal development of the vascular tunics, overgrowth of the intimas, reduplications or absence of the elastica interna, and variable thicknesses of the media. Thinning of the vascular walls may lead to aneurysmal dilatation. Veins are often thickened (arterialized) due to fibrosis and hyalinization (Fig. 7).

A histological feature emphasized by Cushing and Bailey is the presence between the vessels of the AVM of variable amounts of gliotic brain tissue (9). Neighboring cerebral cortex may show neuron loss and astrogliosis. Some degree of subcortical demyelination is usually present.

The occurrence of separate single or multiple intracranial "berry" aneurysms in patients with AVMs was reported by Anderson and Blackwood (2). Numerous additional examples of this association have been described. In most of these cases

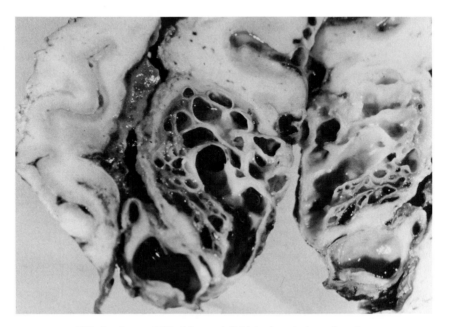

FIG. 6. Large AVM of the occipital lobe (surgical specimen).

the aneurysms and the AVMs were in the same arterial distribution. We have examined the brain of a 35-year-old man who died after a sudden subarachnoid hemorrhage from an intracranial "berry" aneurysm in the initial portion of the right subcallosal artery and who was also found to have an AVM in the distal distribution of the same vessel lying on the posterior portion of the cingulate gyrus (Fig. 8). Anderson and Blackwood (2) considered that these two lesions—aneurysm and AVM—arise independently.

Hirano and Solomon (11), Montoya et al. (19), and Long et al. (15) have reported the association of AVMs of the brain with multiple congenital cardiac defects. AVMs may also occur in infants who have an aneurysm of the vein of Galen.

CRYPTIC VASCULAR HAMARTOMAS

Under this designation Crawford and Russell (8) described small arteriovenous and venous hamartomas which are clinically silent but are significant as a possible cause of spontaneous intracerebral hemorrhage.

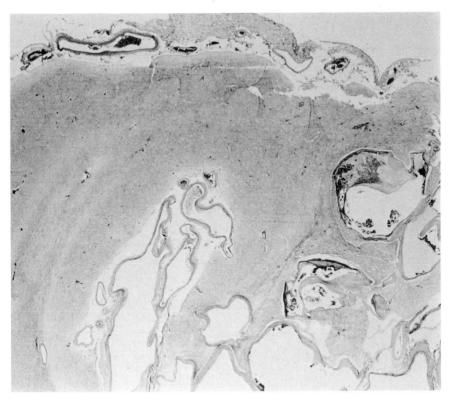

FIG. 7. Photomicrograph of an AVM showing variations in vessel caliber and type with gliotic intervening neural tissue (Trichrome, ×90).

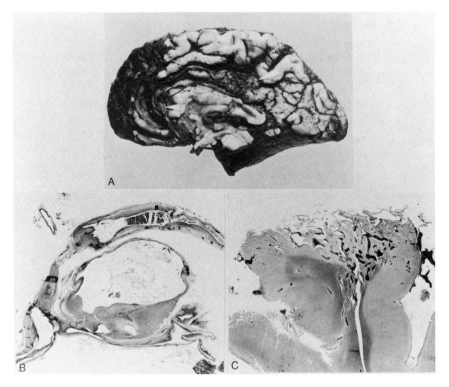

FIG. 8. Association of an intracranial aneurysm with an AVM in the same vascular distribution. **A:** Medial aspect of right cerebral hemisphere showing both vascular lesions; **B:** Photomicrograph of aneurysm of supracallosal artery (H and E, ×5); **C:** Arteriovenous malformation of the cingulate gyrus (H and E, ×5).

These "cryptic" angiomas tend to occur in younger individuals. In some cases of intracerebral hemorrhage, remnants of an angioma are found near the edge of the hematoma or within it. In others, evidence of an angioma may elude the observer, despite special care taken to find it. The clinical importance of these "cryptic" angiomas is that they may cause a sudden fatal brain hemorrhage whose etiology is never identified. McCormick and Nofzinger reviewed this subject and reported 48 cases (17).

REFERENCES

1. Alexander, G. L., and Norman, R. M. (1960): *The Sturge–Weber Syndrome.* Wright, Bristol.
2. Anderson, R. McD., and Blackwood, W. (1959): The association of arteriovenous angioma and saccular aneurysm of the arteries of the brain. *J. Pathol. Bacteriol.,* 77:101.
3. Bergstrand, H., Olivecrona, H., and Tönnis, W. (1936): *Gefässmissbildungen und Gefässgeschwülste des Gehirns.* G. Thieme, Leipzig.
4. Bergstrand, H. (1936): On the classification of the haemangiomatous tumours and malformations of the central nervous system. *Acta. Pathol. Microbiol. Scand. [Suppl.],* 26:89–95.
5. Berry, R. G., Alpers, B. S., White, J. C. (1966): In: *Cerebro Vascular Disease,* edited by C. H. Millikan. Williams and Wilkins, Baltimore.

6. Courville, C. B. (1945): *Pathology of the Central Nervous System*, Second Edition. Pacific Press Pub. Assoc., Mountain View, California.
7. Courville, C. B. (1957): Encephalic lesions in hereditary hemorrhagic telangiectasis (Rendu–Osler–Weber disease). *Bull. Los Angeles Neurol. Soc.*, 22:28–35.
8. Crawford, J. V., and Russell, D. S. (1959): Cryptic arteriovenous hamartomas of brain. *J. Neurol. Neurosurg. Psychiatry*, 19:1–11.
9. Cushing, H., and Bailey, P. (1928): *Tumors Arising from the Blood Vessels of the Brain*. Charles C. Thomas, Springfield, Illinois.
10. Heffner, R. R., Jr., and Solitaire, G. B. (1969): Hereditary hemorrhagic telangiectasia: Neuropathological observations. *J. Neurol. Neurosurg. Psychiatry*, 31:604–608.
11. Hirano, A., and Solomon, S. (1960): Arteriovenous aneurysm of the vein of Galen. *Arch. Neurol.*, 3:589–593.
12. Jellinger, K. (1975): The morphology of centrally situated angiomas. In: *Cerebral Angiomas*, edited by H. W. Pia, J. R. W. Gleave, E. Grote, and J. Zierski, pp. 9–17. Springer-Verlag, Berlin.
13. Kalischer, S. (1897): Demonstration des Gehirns eines Kindes mit Teleangiectasie der linksseitigen Gesicht–Skopfhaut und Hirnoberfläche. *Berl. Klin. Wochenschrift*, 34:1059.
14. Krayenbühl, H., and Yasargil, M. G. (1972): Klinik der Gefässmissbildungen und Gefässfisteln. In: *Der Hirnkreislauf*, edited by H. Gänshirt, pp. 465–511. G. Thieme, Stuttgart.
15. Long, D. M., Seljeskeg, E. L., Chou, S. N., and French, L. A. (1974): Giant arteriovenous malformations of infancy and childhood. *J. Neurosurg.*, 40:304–312.
16. McCormick, W. F. (1966): The pathology of vascular ("arteriovenous") malformations. *J. Neurosurg.*, 24:807–816.
17. McCormick, W. F., and Nofzinger, J. D. (1966): "Cryptic" vascular malformations of the central nervous system. *J. Neurosurg.*, 24:865–875.
18. McCormick, W. F., Hardman, J. M., and Boulter, T. R. (1968): Vascular malformations ("angiomas") of the brain with special reference to those occurring in the posterior fossa. *J. Neurosurg.*, 38:241–251.
19. Montoya, G., Dohn, D. F., and Messer, R. D. (1971): Malformations of the vein of Galen as a cause of heart failure and hydrocephalus in infants. *Neurology (Minneap.)*, 21:1054–1058.
20. Noran, H. H. (1943): Intracranial vascular tumors and malformations. *Arch. Pathol.*, 39:393–416.
21. Olivecrona, H., and Ladenheim, J. (1957): *Congenital Arteriovenous Aneurysms of the Carotid and Vertebral Arterial Systems*. Springer-Verlag, Berlin.
22. Perret, G., and Nishioka, H. (1966): Arteriovenous malformations. An analysis of 545 cases of cranio–cerebral arteriovenous malformations and fistulae reported to the Cooperative Study. *J. Neurosurg.*, 25:467–490.
23. Russell, D. S. (1931): Discussion on vascular tumors of the brain and spinal cord. *Proc. R. Soc. Med.*, 24:383.
24. Russell, D. S., and Rubinstein, J. J. (1977): *Pathology of Tumors of the Nervous System*, Fourth Edition. E. Arnold, London.
25. Sabin, F. R. (1917): Preliminary note on the differentiation of angioblasts and the method by which they produce blood vessels, blood plasma, and red blood cells as seen in the living chick. *Anat. Rec.*, 13:199–205.
26. Sahs, A. L., Perret, G. E., Locksley, H. B., and Nishioka, H. (1969): *Intracranial Aneurysms and Subarachnoid Hemorrhage. A Cooperative Study*. J. B. Lippincott, Philadelphia.
27. Streeter, G. L. (1918): The developmental alterations in the vascular system of the brain of human embryo. *Carnegie Publications*, No. 271, pp. 5–38.
28. Sturge, W. A. (1879): A case of partial epilepsy, apparently due to a lesion of one of the vasomotor centers of the brain. *Trans. Clin. Soc. Lond.*, 162–167.
29. Unna, P. G. (1896): *Histopathology of Diseases of the Skin* (Translation) Edinburgh.
30. Van Bogaert, L. (1950): Pathologie des angiomatoses. *Acta Neurol. Psychiatr. Belg.*, 50:525–610.
31. Virchow, R. (1863): *Die krankhaften Geschwülste* Bd. 3, pp. 306–496. Berlin.
32. Weber, F. P. (1922): Right-sided hemihypotrophy resulting from right-sided congenital spastic Hemiplegia with a morbid condition of the left side of the brain, revealed by radiograms. *J. Neurol. Psychopath.*, 3:134–139.
33. Wyburn–Mason, R. (1943): *The Vascular Abnormalities and Tumours of the Spinal Cord and Its Membranes*. Kimpton, London.
34. Wyburn–Mason, R. (1943): Anteriovenous aneurysm of midbrain and retina, facial naevi, and mental changes. *Brain*, 66:163–203.

Vascular Malformations, edited by
R.R. Smith, A. Haerer and W.F. Russell.
Raven Press, New York © 1982.

Radiographic Features of Vascular Malformations

P. S. Holla, W. F. Russell, R. R. Smith, and W. M. Flowers

Departments of Neurosurgery and Radiology, University of Mississippi Medical Center, Jackson, Mississippi 39216

The first arteriovenous malformation (AVM) of the brain was described by Luschka in 1854. However, definitive preoperative diagnosis could not be made until the development of cerebral angiography by Moniz in 1929. In 1928, Dandy (7) described eight cases and reviewed literature pertinent to the subject. It was clearly demonstrated that nearly one-half of all patients harboring these malformations seek medical attention for reasons other than bleeding. The definitive diagnosis in these cases must rest on the neuroradiological features. In the past 50 years, technology has advanced enormously, and during this interval the radiological findings associated with arteriovenous malformations have been amply described. The present report reviews the literature and presents the current state of the art.

SKULL X-RAYS

The earliest recorded references to radiographic findings must be attributed to Dandy (7), who noted that "the Roentgen ray evidence as in one of the cases which I have reported may, unaided, be sufficient in diagnosis. The presence of calcified shadows, in the circles or whorls, is, I believe, almost pathognomonic of vascular degeneration. When taken in conjunction with clinical data, the diagnosis should be unequivocal." Excellent reviews were published by Rumbaugh and Potts (36), who outlined the following significant radiographic areas of interest: (a) Abnormal calcifications; (b) atrophy and hypertrophy of the skull; (c) enlargement of foramina; (d) enlargement of vascular grooves; (e) changes secondary to mass effect.

The calcifications associated with AVMs may be linear, circumlinear, in the form of parallel lines, punctate, circular, or irregular (Fig. 1). Although calcification was not a common occurrence in the series by Newton and Potts (28), others have described calcific-like densities in up to 30% of cases. With the exception of the Sturge-Weber syndrome and the vein of Galen malformation, these calcifications cannot be distinguished from those occurring with aneurysms or tumors. At times, they appear very faint and only become obvious on computerized tomographic (CT) scan.

Erosion of the skull with AVMs is well known and was originally described by Dandy (7) in 1928. In some of his cases, calvarial thinning, obvious at operation, had been overlooked on routine admission roentgenograms. Rumbaugh and Potts (36) also called attention to erosion of the inner table of the calvarium of patients harboring malformations. Reduction in the size of the hemicranium ipsilateral to

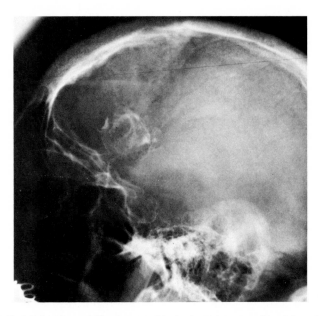

FIG. 1. Calcified AVM. The calcification noted in the frontal area on this plain radiograph has a whorled configuration sometimes seen with AVMs. Although the patient proved to have an AVM on subsequent angiogram, other lesions, especially neoplasms, must be considered in the differential diagnosis.

the AVM was also noted, and perhaps this finding was related to the cerebral hemiatrophy which begins in early childhood (36). In contrast, thickening of the cranial vault has also been noted (36). Analogies have been drawn between skull hypertrophy and the localized gigantism seen in patients with fistulas of the extremities, although it may result from ipsilateral cortical atrophy. Both increased and decreased hemicranial volume have been associated with hypertrophy of the cranium in the Sturge-Weber syndrome (9). Hemangioma of the skull (Fig. 2) associated with intracranial angioma has also been reported (37).

Since vascular malformations lead to increased cardiac output and decreased resistance, there is, as a consequence, a substantial increase in blood flow through the main nutrient vessels of most malformations. Both dilatation and elongation of these feeding arteries follow and, predictably, the foramina through which these vessels enter and exit from the skull enlarge proportionately. Although there is normally considerable variation in the size of the carotid canal, unilateral and bilateral enlargement has been described with malformations (36). Asymmetry has greater significance than absolute measurements and suggests the presence of a malformation. Unilateral and bilateral erosion of the floor of the sella has been described secondary to carotid artery dilatation. Some cases simulate intrasellar tumors, whereas in others the anterior clinoid processes become elevated, mimicking a parasellar mass. In malformations of the vertebrobasilar system, enlargement of the foramina transversaria, deepening of the groove on the lateral mass of the atlas, or enlargement of the arcuate foramina have been described (15). Basilar views of the skull may show enlargement of the jugular fossa, but again, because of variability in normals, gross asymmetry is more helpful than absolute findings (15). If the malformation is supplied by external carotid feeders or drains into the extracranial venous circulation, enlarged emissary foramina may also be observed.

The grooves made by both arterial and venous channels may be affected. Normally, there is considerable variation in the size of the venous channels and hence, enlargement should be interpreted with caution. It is also well known that meningiomas and other neoplasms produce similar changes. Enlargement of the middle meningial groove, particularly along its posterior branch is often noticed with dural malformations about the mastoid process (Fig. 3).

Gross enlargement of the transverse sinus has been reported with an AVM of the posterior cranial fossa (4).

Unless hemorrhage has occurred, displacement of midline structures is extremely unusual. Rumbaugh and Potts (36) reported displacement of the calcified pineal or choroid plexus in 14% of their cases. In some of these there was an associated hematoma, but a shift can occur primarily when large malformations act as mass lesions.

AIR STUDIES

Long before the safety and merits of cerebral angiography were established, the only radiological method available was air ventriculography. Dandy (7) stressed the importance of this tool in defining the presence and the character of an intracranial mass lesion. Although the ventriculogram rarely leads to a direct diagnosis of a malformation, deformity of the ventricles raises the question of an intracranial mass. Association of a malformation with hydrocephalus has been long recognized, and the ventriculogram assists in localization of the obstruction. Occasionally, dilated feeding arteries and draining veins may be recognized by the distortion of sulci through which the enlarged blood vessels course (25).

RADIONUCLIDE STUDIES

Many early and significant observations were made with diagnostic isotopes that produced a relatively low-information density compared to the present isotope of choice, technetium-99m, or one of its compounds. Early successful investigations also used the rectilinear scanner, which has been virtually replaced by the scintillation camera for all brain-scanning studies. Over the past 10 or 15 years, radionuclide studies of the brain have undergone remarkable technical progress. The medical literature documents this dramatic change from relatively primitive techniques. Reports by Meschan et al. (26), Landman and Ross (21), Maynard et al. (24), Rosenthall (35), Morrison et al. (27), Binet and Loken (2), and Gates et al. (11) illustrate this progress.

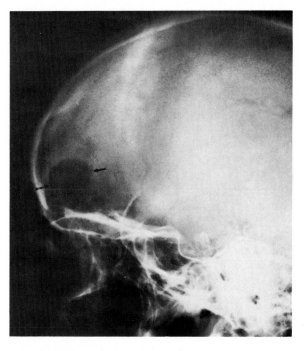

FIG. 2. Hemangioma of the calvarium. **A:** A well-defined lucent erosion in the frontal bone is demonstrated. Note the faint spicules radiating to the periphery from the central portion of the lesion typical of this lesion.

Detection rates have varied from about 50% of the lesions to as high as 100%. The two most important variables appear to be the size of the lesion (38) and the sophistication of the scanning process. Nevertheless, the two basic reasons why most intracranial lesions can be demonstrated by scanning procedures remain the same; either there is more radioactive blood in the lesion than in the surrounding tissues, or there is an abnormal blood–brain barrier.

DYNAMIC RADIONUCLIDE STUDIES

The scintillation camera allows the production of rapid serial films of the initial passage of a radioactive bolus through the brain. The result is analogous to a low-resolution angiogram. Unless the site of the lesion is known in advance, the anterior view is used. A dose of 20 mCi technetium-99m is injected as a very rapid bolus. The AVM produces a striking and characteristic scan series. There is rapid appearance and then rapid disappearance of increased activity as the radioactive bolus passes through the abnormal vessels (Fig. 4). During the initial passage, negligible amounts of blood cross the blood–brain barrier. Maynard et al. (24) and Gates et al. (11) have shown that the only abnormality on the entire study might be seen at

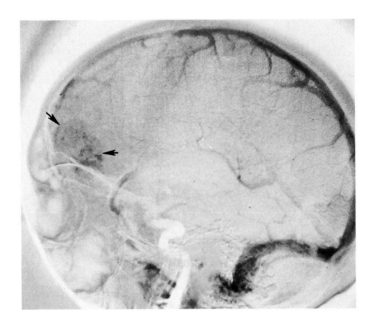

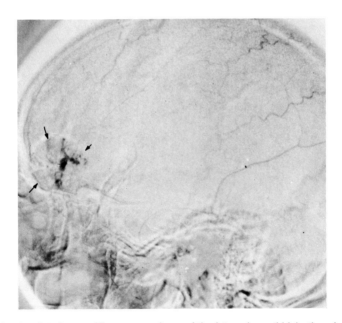

FIG. 2B (top): Arteriogram: The venous phase of the internal carotid injection showed puddling of contrast within the lesion. **C (bottom):** The hemangioma also had external carotid supply demonstrated by contrast collections on late phase of the external carotid injection.

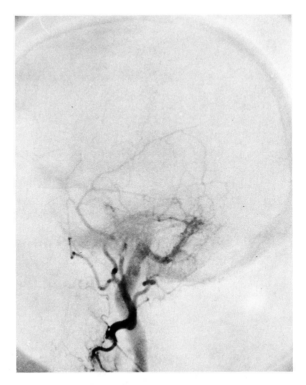

FIG. 3. Dural AVM. External carotid arteriogram (lateral view) shows a pure dural AVM draining into the sigmoid sinus supplied by branches of the posterior division of the middle meningeal artery, the posterior auricular artery, and the occipital artery.

this time. At times, however, delayed static views will show a circumscribed focal lesion that has a striking correlation with the flow study.

Tully et al. (40) and Curl et al. (6) reported diagnosing carotid cavernous fistula on flow studies. They have emphasized its role in evaluation of treatment, particularly in the early postoperative periods.

COMPUTER ANALYSIS OF RADIONUCLIDE SCANS

Binet and Loken (2) demonstrated that computer analysis of brain uptake shows a remarkable difference in the amount of radioactive tracer within the lesion as compared with the normal brain. Recently, Gates et al. (11) reported a 100% detection of AVMs in 9 children with the use of combinations of static, dynamic, and computer-processed images. Two of these AVMs were missed by CT scans. This may be related to the timing of CT scan and or lack of breakdown of the blood–brain barrier.

VALUE OF RADIONUCLIDE STUDIES

Modern static, dynamic, and computer-processed radionuclide studies may well prove to be the most effective screening method for detecting the presence of an AVM because of accuracy and lower cost. The AVM produces a very characteristic pattern on dynamic imaging. Static (Fig. 4D) and dynamic studies are complementary in many ways. The rapid appearance and disappearance of the lesion in the dynamic study points toward vascular malformations. Highly vascular tumors such as meningiomas and malignant gliomas, in contrast, may show a rapid accumulation of radioactivity on the flow study but with much less rapid washout. Angiography may prove to be the definitive procedure, but radionuclide studies do not require anesthesia, heavy sedation, or iodinated contrast agents.

ANGIOGRAPHY

Arteriography, to quote Pool (31) is "the key test for the diagnosis of an arteriovenous malformation." The uses of angiography in the evaluation of patients with suspected vascular malformations are multiple: (a) to confirm the diagnosis; (b) to localize the fistula exactly; (c) to map feeding arteries and draining veins; and (d) to study the feasibility of nonsurgical therapeutic procedures, such as embolization.

When angiography is indicated, the maximum information of finest detail will be demanded, and it should only be performed by those with considerable experience, in consultation with the surgeon. Otherwise, the CT scan serves a satisfactory function merely to document the presence of the lesion. Arteriography, of course, is always indicated when the cause of subarachnoid hemorrhage has not been established by noninvasive modalities. Even after the complete study, if the lesion is not apparent, selective external carotid studies are needed in the suspicious case. Intracranial AVMs exclusively fed by the external carotid artery are not rarities (5,33) (Fig. 3). According to Parkinson and Bachers (30), "the most dramatic, but the least helpful films are those showing the explosion of contrast medium billowing out into the draining veins." A smaller volume of contrast material provides more information, avoiding the obscuration of details caused by the explosion. The advantage of rapid simultaneous biplane serial angiography in intracranial AVMs cannot be overemphasized (29). The cassette changer should start as soon as injection starts, and exposure should continue at the rate of 5 to 6 per sec in order to map out the final feeding arteries and fistula phase.

Although it is generally recognized that large symptomatic intracranial vascular malformations are nearly always demonstrated by angiography, the same is definitely not true for the smaller vascular malformations which are occasionally found by the unsuspecting surgeon or by the pathologist (Fig. 5). Only a few large vascular malformations have escaped detection by serial angiography (17), and the failure in these cases has been attributed to: (a) abnormally rapid or slow circulation

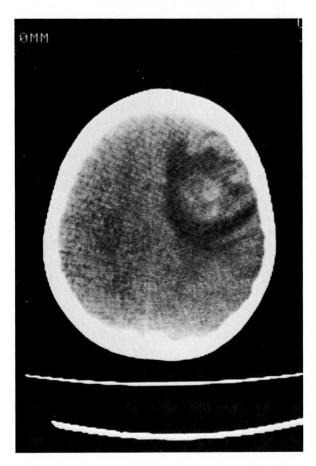

FIG. 4A. Intracerebral hemorrhage. A CT scan on this 7-year-old child was obtained because of apparent head trauma. A fronto-parietal mass lesion of mixed density is demonstrated.

time; (b) partial or complete thrombosis of a malformation; (c) failure to opacify the appropriate feeding artery by not doing complete studies; and (d) certain malformations such as cavernous angiomas may be totally isolated from the main vascular supply of the brain.

The cavernous hemangioma may be angiographically silent (Fig. 6). Prolonged injection with delayed film sequence concentrates the venous phase of the circulation and aids in the demonstration of these malformations (3,8,34).

The telangiectatic lesion also requires special techniques, such as subtraction, magnification, and angiotomography to outline the lesion accurately and to assist the surgeon in planning resection. Intravenous radioangiography may have a role in the near future, reducing the inherent risk associated with arteriography, particularly in older patients.

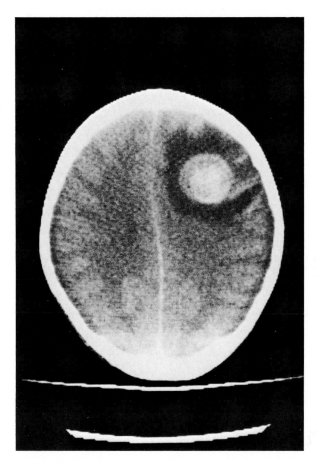

FIG. 4B. The postcontrast scan shows a well-defined rounded lesion of increased density with rim enhancement and considerable surrounding edema. Brain tumor was considered to be the main differential possibility.

COMPUTERIZED AXIAL TOMOGRAPHY

With the development of computerized tomography, further refinement of noninvasive diagnostic methodology became available. The typical appearance of a cerebral AVM on the CT scan is characterized by discrete areas of high density compared to the density of the surrounding brain (32) (Fig. 7). The increased density may be accounted for by (a) mural calcification within the walls of the vessels (Fig. 8), (b) occurrence of subclinical hemorrhage, and (c) calcification or gliosis of the intervening brain tissue. Terbrugge et al. (41) noted that these high-density areas may have absorption coefficients which range from 50 to 100 + Hounsefield units.

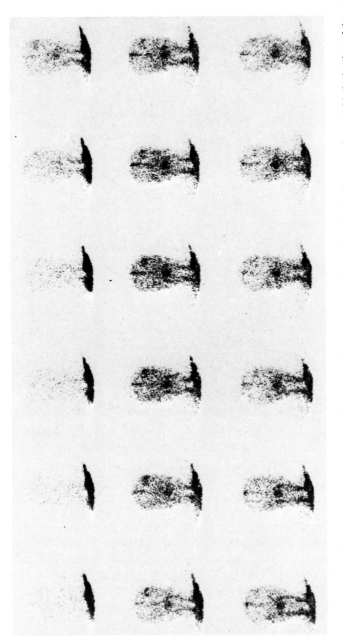

Fig. 4C. The radionuclide flow study demonstrates rapid accumulation of radioactivity overlying the lesion as well as rapid dissipation of the activity on subsequent frames. Such a pattern is virtually diagnostic of AVM. Some highly vascular tumors or arteriovenous fistulas can, however, mimic this flow pattern.

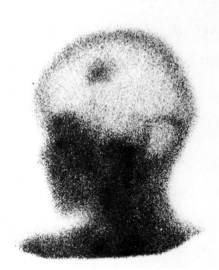

FIG. 4D. The static nuclide scan shows a nonspecific pattern. The lesion is noted to be in the left frontal lobe, but there are no features distinguishing it from tumor, stroke, abscess, or hematoma. This static scan adds little which the CT scan has not already provided. The flow study, on the other hand, contributed invaluable information which compelled further work-up.

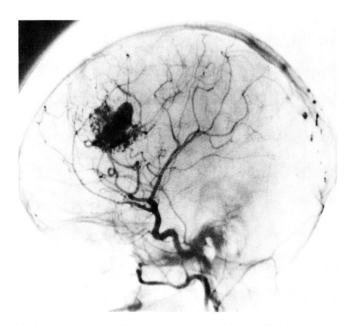

FIG. 4E. Arteriography confirms the diagnosis of an AVM supplied by anterior and middle cerebral feeders. Note the nidus of abnormal vessels uniformly arranged and benign in appearance. Large early draining veins such as the one seen overlying the nidus are typical for AVMs.

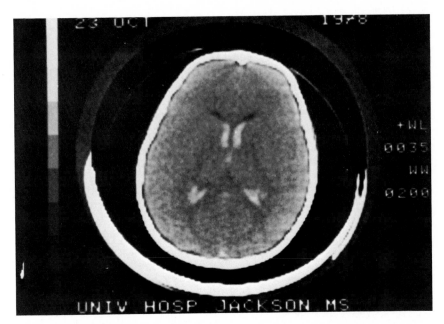

FIG. 5. Cryptic AVM. **A:** A CT brain scan was obtained because of spontaneous subarachnoid hemorrhage revealing intraventricular hemorrhage. Note the small extraventricular collection of blood just lateral to the atrium of the right lateral ventricle.

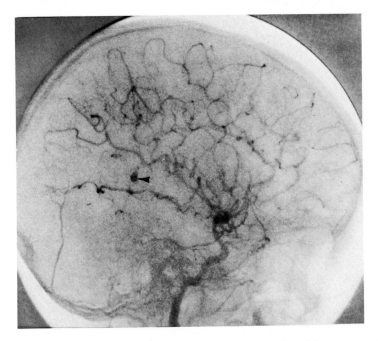

FIG. 5B. Complete angiography was normal except for the small puddle of contrast in the parietal area in the late arterial phase (arrowhead). This finding was believed sufficient for the diagnosis of cryptic AVM, the major portion of the lesion probably having obliterated itself during the hemorrhage.

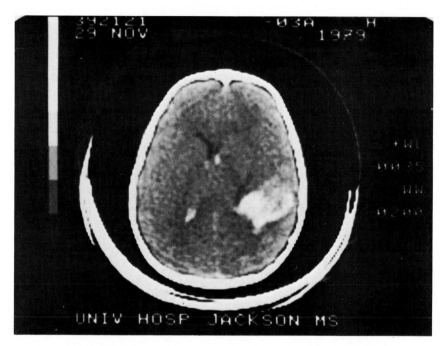

FIG. 5C. One year later, the patient returned with a second bleeding episode. The CT scan at this time revealed a large posterior temporal lobe hematoma with extension into the ventricular system. Surgical evacuation of the hematoma and AVM remnants was performed, and pathologic confirmation was obtained. The patient recovered completely and was discharged.

The low-density areas immediately adjacent to the malformation are probably due to cerebral atrophy. Generalized enlargement of the ventricles, dilatation of the ipsilateral ventricle, focal mass effect (22), and atrophy of or hypertrophy of the hemicranium (19) provide indirect evidence for the presence of a malformation. A word of caution concerning nonenhanced studies is in order, since they may be completely normal in almost one-fourth of all cases in which the lesion can be demonstrated angiographically.

Considering the low sensitivity of the routine CT scans for vascular malformations, contrast enhancement should be employed in every case in which a lesion is suspected. High-density areas seen on plain scans, if due to vascular malformations, are exaggerated by enhancement, and diagnostic accuracy rates of over 90% have been reported (16,18). Enhancement following injection of iodinated material is due to both intra- and extravascular accumulation (12). Bergstrom et al. (1) calculated that at an iodine level of 4 mg/ml, vessels as small as 1.5 mm can be defined. However, this sensitivity can probably never be improved upon, and further delineation of blood vessels smaller than 1.5 mm must remain in the domain of angiography.

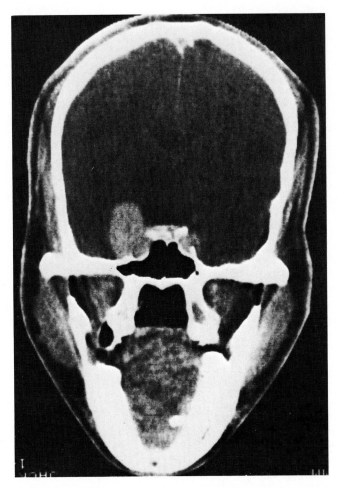

FIG. 6. Cavernoma. This contrast-enhanced CT scan cut in the coronal plane reveals a well-defined, homogeneously enhanced, parasellar lesion. Aneurysm and meningioma were considered the main differential possibilities until the normal arteriogram ruled out aneurysm and made meningioma less likely. A prolonged injection angiogram with delayed film sequence might have provided sufficient clues to make the correct diagnosis of cavernoma.

The contrast-enhanced scan provides visualization of large feeding arteries and draining veins, making definitive diagnosis possible (Fig. 7B). There is some evidence that the CT scan with contrast exceeds the overall effectiveness of angiography in defining cavernous hemangiomas and cryptic vascular malformations (20,39). It must be recognized, however, that vascular malformations can be mistaken for gliomas (10), infarction (18) (Fig. 7B), and vice versa. The absence of surrounding edema and mass effect should favor diagnosis of the vascular lesion.

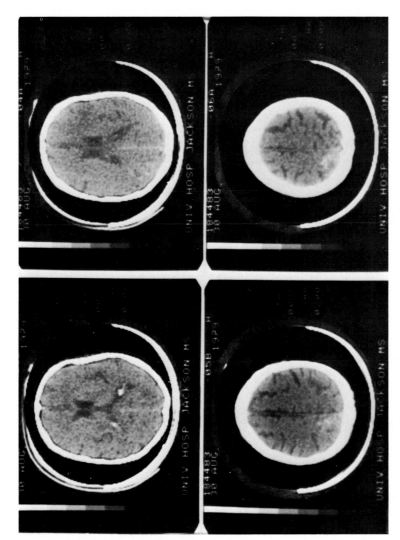

FIG. 7. AVM parietal lobe. **A:** CT scan: Focal areas of increased density are noted in the left parietal lobe. The higher cuts reveal calcification not appreciable on plain skull radiographs even in retrospect. No mass effect is evident.

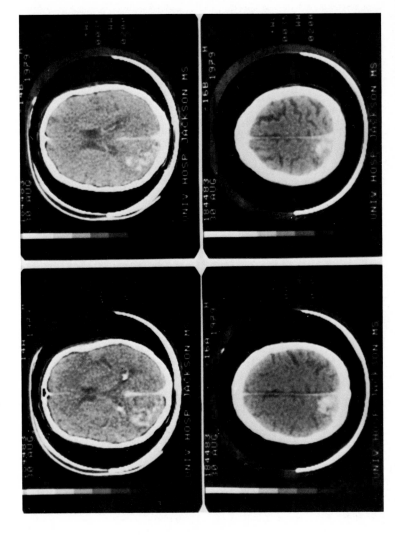

FIG. 7B. Following contrast, the appearance of tubular or vermiform areas of enhancement strongly suggests the diagnosis of AVM. Sometimes "gyral enhancement" in patients with recent cerebral infarction may have a similar scan pattern, but the presence of calcification on plain scan excludes this possibility.

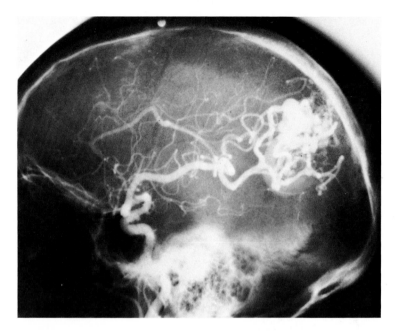

FIG. 7C. The arteriogram confirms the diagnosis and demonstrates the left middle cerebral artery to be the predominant supply.

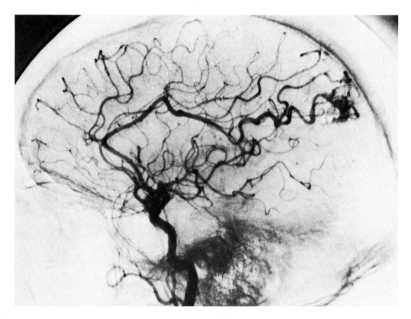

FIG. 7D. The contralateral carotid injection opacifies both anterior cerebral arteries, revealing the presence of additional supply to the AVM from the left anterior cerebral group.

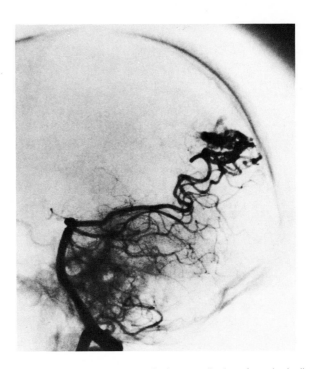

FIG. 7E. The vertebral injection documents further contributions from the ipsilateral posterior cerebral group.

For the first time, utilizing computed tomography, the intraventricular clot may be visualized (Fig. 5). Intraparenchymal hematomas (Figs. 4A and 5C), as well as subarachnoid hemorrhage (23), are also easily localized with this method. The hematomas most likely to be misinterpreted, however, are those associated with angiomas and neoplasms (13). The hemorrhage from AVMs can usually be differentiated from the hypertensive hemorrhage on the basis of the location on computerized scan. Hemorrhage from aneurysms may be seen in the septum pellucidum, ventricles, interhemispheric region, basal cisterns, and along the sylvian fissure. Hypertensive hemorrhages are commonly found in the vicinity of basal ganglia, thalamus, and cerebellum. Any cortical hemorrhage may be due to AVM or tumor (13) (Fig. 4). It has been shown that even in the presence of bleeding, hematomas due to AVM often show abnormal vascular enhancement. Hence, there is definite need for contrast enhancement study in all atypical intraparenchymal bleeds (14). Focal hematomas immediately adjacent to a ventricular wall and bulging into the ventricular cavity are especially suggestive of vascular malformations (18).

Another important role that CT has assumed is differentiating which of multiple vascular lesions demonstrated by arteriography has actually bled. This problem arises when concurrent AVM and aneurysm or multiple aneurysms are present. Computerized tomography usually shows fresh blood adjacent to the affected lesion (Fig. 9).

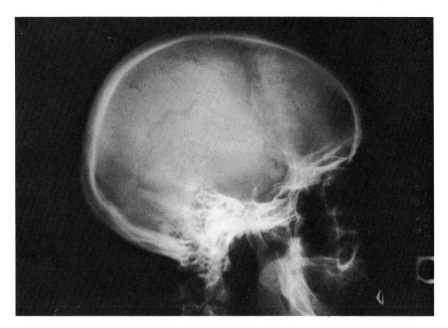

FIG. 8. Variant of vein of Galen aneurysm. **A:** Plain skull radiograph shows "egg-shell" type calcification. The differential diagnosis includes vein of Galen aneurysm and pineal area neoplasm.

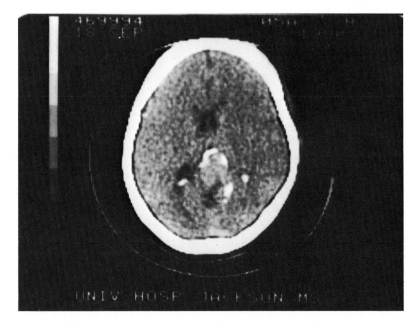

FIG. 8B. Contrast-enhanced CT scan demonstrates a homogeneously enhancing pineal area lesion with rim calcification. There is no significant hydrocephalus, a factor against neoplasm which usually obstructs the ventricular system in this strategic location.

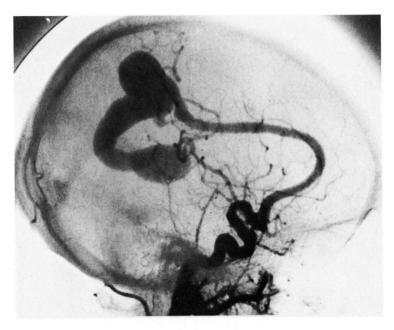

FIG. 8C. The arteriogram shows a markedly dilated anterior cerebral artery which empties into an enlarged venous structure in the parasagittal parietal lobe, which subsequently drains into the bulbous calcified vein of Galen. A minor contribution to the AVM is noted from the middle cerebral group. No definitive nidus is identified.

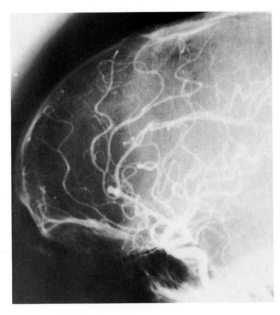

FIG. 9A. Multiple lesions. Arteriogram done because of subarachnoid hemorrhage in this patient showed the presence of an aneurysm of the anterior cerebral artery arising at its bifurcation between the pericallosal and callosomarginal arteries.

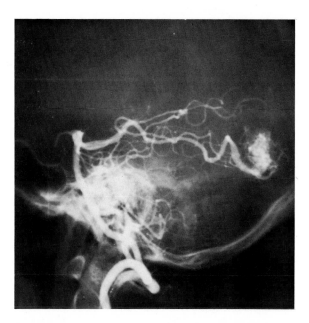

FIG. 9B. Multiple lesions (same patient as Fig. 9A). The vertebral injection showed an occipital lobe AVM supplied by the posterior cerebral artery. The association of the two lesions is known to occur in a small percentage of cases, and subarachnoid hemorrhage can be a complication of either. Although the angiogram did not establish which one of these lesions bled, a small parenchymal hematoma surrounding and thus implicating the aneurysm was found on CT scan.

Finally, the computerized scan is an excellent tool for continued evaluation, especially in the case of the deteriorating patient or in those seriously ill from hemorrhage. Even angiography may provide insufficient information to define the mechanisms of hemorrhage and precisely localize the anatomical structures involved. The computerized scan, however, reliably records hydrocephalus and often points to the underlying pathology such as aqueductal obstruction or a clot within the fourth ventricle. Recurrent or continued bleedings may be recorded by the computerized scan, and any surrounding infarction may be visualized.

REFERENCES

1. Bergstrom, M., Riding, M., and Greitz, T. (1976): The limitations of definition of blood vessels with computer intravenous angiography. *Neuroradiology*, 11:35–40.
2. Binet, E. F., and Loken, M. K. (1970): Scintiangiography of cerebral arteriovenous malformations and aneurysms. *Am. J. Roetgenol.*, 109:707–713.
3. Bogren, H., Svalander, C., and Wickbom, I. (1970): Angiography in intracranial cavernous hemangiomas. *Acta Radiol. [Diagn.] (Stockh.)*, 10:81–89.
4. Cash, M. D., McGinnis, K. D., and Knighton, R. S. (1966): Posterior fossa arteriovenous aneurysm with calvarial change. *Radiology*, 86:529–531.
5. Ciminello, V. J., and Sachs, E., Jr. (1962): Arteriovenous malformations of the posterior fossa. *J. Neurosurg.*, 19:602–604.
6. Curl, F. D., Harbert, J. C., and Lussenhop, A. D. (1972): Radionuclide cerebral angiography in a case of bilateral carotid cavernous fistula. *Radiology*, 102:391–392.

7. Dandy, W. E. (1928): Arteriovenous aneurysm of the brain. *Arch. Surg.*, 17:190–243.
8. Diamond, C., Torvik, A., and Amundsen, P. (1976): Angiographic diagnosis of teleangiectases with cavernous angioma of the posterior fossa. *Acta Radiol. [Diagn.] (Stockh.)*, 17:281–287.
9. Enzmann, D. R., Hayward, R. W., Norman, D., and Dunn, R. P. (1977): Cranial computed tomographic scan appearance of Sturge–Weber disease. Unusual presentation. *Radiology*, 122:721–724.
10. Foy, P. M., Lozada, L., and Shaw, M. D. (1981): Vascular malformation simulating a glioma on computed tomography. *J. Neurosurg.*, 54:125–127.
11. Gates, G. F., Fishman, L. S., and Segall, H. D. (1978): Scintigraphic detection of congenital intracranial vascular malformations. *J. Nucl. Med.*, 19:235–244.
12. Hatam, A., Bergvall, U., Lewander, R., Larsson, S., and Lind, M. (1975): Contrast medium enhancement with time in computer tomography. *Acta Radiol.*, 346:63–81.
13. Hayward, R. D., and O'Reilly, G. V. A. (1976): Intracranial hemorrhage: Accuracy of computerized transverse axial scanning in predicting the underlying etiology. *Lancet*, 1:1–4.
14. Hayward, R. D. (1976): Intracranial arteriovenous malformations. *J. Neurol. Neurosurg. Psychiatry*, 39:1027–1033.
15. Hoare, R. D. (1953): Arteriovenous aneurysm of the posterior fossa. *Acta Radiol.*, 40:96–102.
16. Jensen, H. P., Klinge, H., Lemke, J., Muhtaroglu, U., and Rautenberg, M. (1980): Computerized tomography in vascular malformations of the brain. *Neurosurg. Rev.*, 3:119–127.
17. Kamarin, R. B., and Buschbaum, H. W. (1965): Large vascular malformations of the brain not visualized by serial angiography. *Arch. Neurol.*, 13:413–420.
18. Kendall, B. E., and Claveria, L. E. (1976): The use of computed axial tomography (CAT) for the diagnosis and management of intracranial angiomas. *Neuroradiol.*, 12:141–160.
19. Kido, D. K., LeMay, M., Han, S. S., and Strand, R. (1979): Diagnosis of cranial asymetries in cerebral arteriovenous malformations. *J. Comp. Assisted Tomography*, 3:221–225.
20. Kramer, R. A., and Wing, D. S. (1977): Computed tomography of angiographically occult cerebral vascular malformations. *Radiology*, 123:649–652.
21. Landman, S., and Ross, P. (1973): Radionuclides in the diagnosis of arteriovenous malformations of the brain. *Radiology*, 108:635–639.
22. Leblanc, R., Ethier, R., and Little, J. R. (1979): Computerized tomography findings in arteriovenous malformations of the brain. *J. Neurosurg.*, 51:765–772.
23. Lim, S. T., and Sage, D. J. (1977): Detection of subarachnoid blood clot and other thin flat structures by computerized tomography. *Radiology*, 123:79–84.
24. Maynard, D. C., Witcofski, R. L., Janeway, R., and Cowan, R. J. (1969): Radioisotope arteriography as an adjunct to the brain scan. *Radiology*, 92:908–912.
25. McRae, D. L., and Valentino, V. (1958): Pneumographic findings in angioma of the brain. *Acta Radiol.*, 50:18–24.
26. Meschan, I., Lytle, W. P., Maynard, D. C., Cowan, R. J., and Janeway, R. (1971): Statistical relationship of brain scans, cervicocranial dynamic studies and cerebral arteriograms. *Radiology*, 100:623–629.
27. Morrison, R. T., Afifi, A. K., Van Allen, M. W., and Evans, T. C. (1965): Scintiencephalography for the detection and localization of non-neoplastic intracranial lesions. *J. Nucl. Med.*, 6:7–15.
28. Newton, T. H., and Potts, D. G. (1974): *Radiology of the Skull and Brain.* Book 4, pp. 2491–2565. C. V. Mosby, St. Louis.
29. Parkinson, D. (1969): Rapid serial simultaneous biplane stereoscopic angiography; an aid in the surgical management of the cerebral arteriovenous malformations. *Clin. Neurosurg.*, 16:170–184.
30. Parkinson, D., and Bachers, G. (1980): Arteriovenous malformations. *J. Neurosurg.*, 53:285–299.
31. Pool, J. L. (1962): Treatment of arteriovenous malformations of the cerebral hemispheres. *J. Neurosurg.*, 19:136–141.
32. Pressman, B. D., Kirkwood, R. J., and Davis, D. O. (1975): Computerized transverse tomography of vascular lesions of the brain. Part 1: Arteriovenous malformations. *Am. J. Roentgenol.*, 124:208–215.
33. Ramamurthy, B., and Balasubramanian, V. (1966): Arteriovenous malformations with a purely external carotid contribution. *J. Neurosurg.*, 25:643–647.
34. Roberson, G. H., Kase, C. S., and Wolpow, E. R. (1974): Telangiectases and cavernous angiomas of the brainstem: "Cryptic" vascular malformations. *Neuroradiol.*, 8:83–89.
35. Rosenthall, L. (1968): Radionuclide diagnosis of arteriovenous malformations with rapid sequence brain scans. *Radiology*, 91:1185–1188.

36. Rumbaugh, C. L., and Potts, G. D. (1966): Skull changes associated with intracranial arteriovenous malformations. *Am. J. Roentgenol.*, 98:525–534.
37. Scheinberg, L., and Elkin, M. (1958): Hemangioma of the skull associated with intracranial angioma. *Neurology (Minneap.)*, 8:650–652.
38. Shishikura, A., DeLand, F. H., and Gilday, D. (1970): Sensitivity of brain scanning in the detection of arteriovenous malformations. *Radiology*, 97:95–98.
39. Terao, H., Hori, T., Matsutani, M., and Okeda, R. (1979): Detection of cryptic vascular malformations by computerized tomography. *J. Neurosurg.*, 51:546–551.
40. Tully, T. E., Shafer, R. B., Reinke, D. B., and Pliego, M. P. (1974): Radionuclide angiography in the diagnosis of carotid cavernous sinus fistula. *J. Nucl. Med.*, 15:797–800.
41. Terbrugge, K., Scotti, G., Ethier, R., Melancon, D., Tchang, S., and Milner, C. (1977): Computed tomography in intracranial arteriovenous malformations. *Radiology*, 122:703–705.

examination. The present series contains 20 cases in which no causes could be identified by any diagnostic method or from operative specimens. The clinical features of those patients were quite similar to those reported by Margolis and others in 1951 (4), shown in the bottom of Fig. 1. Because the etiology of these cases is considered to be unidentified small angiomatous malformations, this patient group was included with the small AVM and angioma group for the present clinical analysis.

Figure 2 shows the left intracranial carotid angiograms of a 10-year-old girl who complained of sudden severe headache. A small-sized AVM with massive intracerebral hematoma is clearly demonstrated in the frontobasal region, and both feeding arteries and draining veins are also distinguished. Typical AVMs showing feeding arteries, draining veins, and the nidus in the angiogram were excluded from the present study, even if their size was as small as shown in this slide.

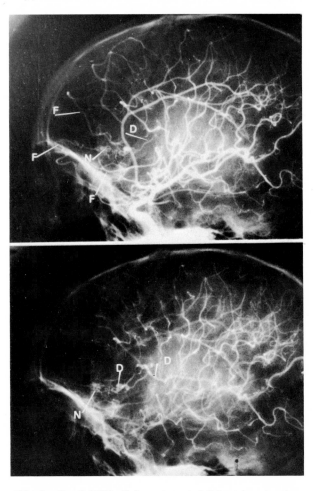

FIG. 2. Small AVM with hematoma in left frontobasal region.

RESULTS

Figure 3 details the age distribution of results of the present series of 46 cases. The open columns in the figure designate patients in whom no vascular anomalies could be found at operation, and the dotted columns indicate those in whom vascular anomalies were verified at operation or by angiography. From a total of 46 cases, 35 were males and 11 females. Although the age of the patients ranged from 4 to 62, and the average age was 31 years, most were observed during the third to fifth decades.

In 25 out of 46 cases, vascular anomalies responsible for bleeding were verified at operation. Histologically (Table 1), 14 cases were AVMs consisting of abnormal arterial and venous vessels separated by gliotic tissue. Three cases were revealed to be cavernous angiomas. They were composed of thin-walled sinusoidal vessels separated by fibrous tissue with no intervening brain parenchyma. The remaining 8 cases were capillary angiomas consisting of small vascular spaces lined by a single layer of endothelium.

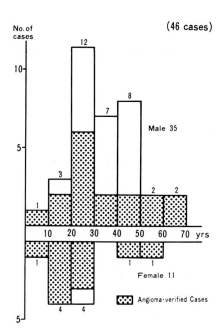

FIG. 3. Age distribution of spontaneous intracranial hemorrhage due to cerebral vascular anomalies and "Unknown causes" (46 cases).

TABLE 1. *Histological diagnosis of vascular anomalies with intracranial hemorrhage (N = 25)*

Vascular anomaly	No. of cases
AVM	14
Cavernous angioma	3
Capillary angioma	8

Characteristic clinical features of these intracerebral hemorrhages were headache of sudden onset, nausea, and vomiting occasionally followed by focal or general convulsive seizures. Usually hemiparesis and disturbance of consciousness developed later within 1 or 2 days. Figure 4 illustrates the carotid angiograms of a 40-year-old man with an interesting clinical course. He had an episode of loss of consciousness associated with a general convulsive seizure 6 years before, and he experienced similar attacks 2 or 3 years later. Five months prior to his admission,

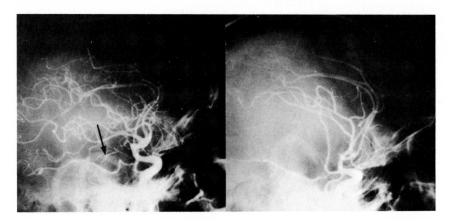

FIG. 4. Angiograms (see text) of a "disappearing" AVM.

he noticed gradual development of right-sided hemianopia and weakness of the extremities on the same side. Left carotid angiogram revealed an abnormal small vascular shadow in the cisternal portion of the anterior choroidal artery. He refused operation and left the hospital. Three days after his discharge, however, he suffered from a sudden severe headache. The following morning he became comatose after a general convulsive seizure and died 2 days later. The right angiogram in Fig. 4 was taken after the last episode of hemorrhage. In addition to a marked shift of the middle cerebral artery, it was noticed that the abnormal vascular shadow had disappeared. This fact suggests, as Russell and others (6) reported, that a small angiomatous malformation could be destroyed at the time of bleeding. It is also suggested that rebleeding is not rare in these conditions.

Table 2 shows the final outcome of cases submitted to surgery. Of 44 patients, 36 were able to work even though some neurological deficits remained. Comparing this operative result to the reported results of hypertensive intracerebral hemorrhages, it is obvious that intracerebral hemorrhage caused by small AVMs and angiomas carries a far better prognosis than hypertensive ones. This may be due to the fact that the favorite site of hemorrhage differs in these disorders, and also may be due to the differences in the source of bleeding. In hypertensive hemorrhage the bleeding occurs in the small arterioles. In small AVMs or angiomas, however, it takes place on the nonarterial side. In the present series, two out of five deaths, nevertheless, were due to rebleeding. It must be stressed that surgery should be

TABLE 2. *Final outcome of cases submitted to surgical treatment (N = 44)*

Outcome	No. of cases
Working	36
Caring for self	3
Died	5

attempted not only to evacuate the hematoma but also to search for and to extirpate the angiomatous malformation.

The recent development of computerized tomography (CT) has brought about changes in the concepts of angiomatous malformations. Table 3 shows the clinical features of our cases admitted after introduction of CT in 1976. It is noticeable that the initial symptoms were not always related to the bleeding. In 8 out of 14 cases the onsets were epileptic attacks including convulsive or psychomotor seizures. This contrasts with the report of McCormick and Nofzinger (5). They reported that epilepsy, commonly found in the classic supratentorial AV malformation, had not been present in their 48 patients with cryptic vascular malformations. In one patient of the present series the mode of onset and the progression of symptoms were very similar to those of a brain tumor. In 3 out of 8 cases with AVM and in 3 out of 5 with cavernous angiomas, diagnosis could be made only by CT. They could not be diagnosed by angiography even with the aid of subtraction or magnification techniques. Recently Becker and others (1) have proposed the name "angiographically occult angioma" for these cases.

COMMENTS

Figure 5 summarizes the clinical significance of AVMs. Most of these vascular anomalies can be diagnosed even before hemorrhage by the use of CT scans. Therefore, it seems necessary to regard these vascular anomalies not only as possible sources of hemorrhage but also as causes of epileptic attacks. The frequency of incidental discovery of these vascular anomalies is increasing with the wider use of CT scans. For those patients with frequent epileptic attacks, surgical intervention may at times be considered for the prevention of such attacks or possible intracranial hemorrhages, especially in patients who have a history of previous intracranial hemorrhages.

It has been our impression from angiograms that most incidentally found vascular anomalies show the characteristic picture of a venous angioma with widespread

TABLE 3. *Intracranial angiomas diagnosed by CT[a]*

Histological diagnosis	Inital symptom			With hematoma	Postive findings in angiography
	Hemorrhage	Epilepsy	Tumor-like		
AVM	8	4	3	1	5/8	5/8
Cavernous angioma	5	1	4		3/5	2/5
Capillary angioma	1		1		1/1	1/1

[a]Fourteen cases diagnosed since 1976.

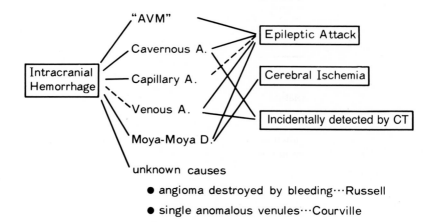

FIG. 5. Clinical significance of cerebral vascular malformations.

medullary veins. Since the risk of bleeding from this type of angioma has been shown to be low, we would like to emphasize the need for careful consideration of surgical indications.

REFERENCES

1. Becker, D. H., Townsend, J. T., Kramer, R. A., and Newton, T. H. (1978): Occult cerebrovascular malformations. A series of histologically verified cases with negative angiography. *Brain*, 102:249–287.
2. Courville, C. B. (1963): Morphology of small vascular malformations of the brain with particular reference to the mechanism of their drainage. *J. Neuropathol. Exp. Neurol.*, 22:274–284.
3. Krayenbuhl, H. A. (1975): The Moya-moya syndrome and the neurosurgeon. *Surg. Neurol.*, 4:353–360.
4. Margolis, G., Odom, G. L., Woodhall, B., and Bloor, B. M. (1951): The role of small angiomatous malformations in the production of intracerebral hematomas. *J. Neurosurg.*, 8:564–575.
5. McCormick, W. F., and Nofzinger, J. D. (1966): "Cryptic" vascular malformations of the central nervous system. *J. Neurosurg.*, 24:865–975.
6. Russell, D. S. (1954): The pathology of intracranial hemorrhage. *Proc. R. Soc. Med.*, 47:689–693.

Vascular Malformations, edited by
R. R. Smith, A. Haerer and W. F. Russell.
Raven Press, New York © 1982.

The Neurosurgical Direct Approach to Cerebral Arteriovenous Malformations

Dwight Parkinson

Department of Surgery, Section of Neurosurgery, The University of Manitoba, Winnipeg, Manitoba R3E0W3

The arteriovenous malformation (AVM) remains, and probably always will be, a formidable challenge to neurological surgeons in spite of all our recent advances in radiology, anesthesia, and instrumentation. Both Cushing and Dandy warned that these lesions be left alone unless they are small and superficial.

The first step in the open surgical approach is the understanding of the pathophysiology. The lack of the interposition of a capillary bed, and hence, the lack of its twin functions, pressure reduction and tissue nutrition, is the basic abnormality. Thus, an artery or arteries flow directly into a vein. The junction, whether single or multiple, may range in diameter from a vessel as large as the carotid down to anything larger than a capillary. From the understanding of this basic pathology, the neurosurgeon has several lessons to remember. First, it is not necessary to pursue the feeding vessels nor the leaving veins beyond their points of attachment to the fistula. Removal or obliteration of the fistula corrects the pathology. Next, the surgeon must remember that any obliteration of the arterial tree proximal to the departure of the final feeding artery can only worsen this cerebral blood supply as the fistula remains to steal from whatever residual collateral is left distal to the occluded site. Obliterating the fistula, however, can only improve the cerebral circulation, provided no additional vessels are occluded. A surgeon can be reassured in the knowledge that he may be as aggressive and as destructive as he wishes within the mass of the fistula with no fear of infarcting any tissue beyond and no fear of destroying functioning tissue within, as the tissue within these abnormal connecting vessels is always glial, other forms of scar tissue, and nonfunctioning neural tissue. The vessels, once they depart to become a fistulous connection, never reconstitute and go on to supply tissue beyond. However, there may be very normal functioning tissue running through the looping tangled approaching arteries and leaving veins, and also there are frequently significant arterial channels running very close to the malformation that must be spared.

The second step in the approach is an adequate angiographic visualization. Particularly with the rapid flow lesions, it is important that the pictures be taken at least as fast as three per second and preferably faster. The cassette changer should be started as soon as, or even before, the injection is given to ensure that the leading edge of the contrast medium is captured as it accelerates with a puff of visualization into and through the first departure of the final feeding artery. The acceleration is due, of course, to the sudden confrontation with a lower bed of resistance. This film is often the most important feature of a single series. It should be emphasized over and over that the actual fistula is frequently very small, and the apparent huge size is due to a combination of multicentric fistulas plus the overshadowing tortuous dilated approaching arteries and departing veins.

The value of stereoscopic views cannot be overemphasized. Any time spent studying the three-dimensional views afforded by stereoscopic angiography is well rewarded at surgery. I doubt if any neurosurgeon has ever thought that he was too well acquainted with the relationship of the fistula to the adjacent feeding arteries, and the arteries going past or the draining veins, once he gets into the exposure. Stereoscopic views may be obtained in two ways. One series may be taken and then the tube shifted and another series taken. This runs a risk that there may be some movement between the two injections. At our institution, we have two off-set tubes that fire alternately, thereby producing a series of stereoscopic views with a single injection. Every odd-numbered film will stereo with every even-numbered film. In this way, the passage of the contrast material can be followed through the lesion with continuous stereoscopic study. At our center, we have an identical unit of double off-set tubes for an AP projection. With these out of synchronization by a few milliseconds and with proper grids, simultaneous AP and lateral serial stereoscopic angiography can be obtained without fogging.

The third step in the approach is to have a plan worked out preoperatively and stick to it at surgery. The plan may be to go as rapidly as possible through the borders of the malformation to get to the final feeding artery. This is probably the best plan when the final feeding arteries are accessible near the surface and where they all come from one direction. Occasionally, with a single draining vein and fairly low flow lesion, the plan might be to ligate and divide the draining vein and then use that as a "handle," gradually mobilizing the lesion dividing the entering arteries. This was advocated by Malis, and we have found it useful on occasions. With large lesions, presenting on the surface as most of them do with another presentation at the surface of the ventricle and, particularly, in cases where there is a considerable porencephaly beneath the lesion as there often is, the plan may be to go through a relatively avascular nonsensitive area of the cortex into the ventricle. By placing a thumb or index finger in the ventricle the surgeon can squeeze the malformation between his thumb and index finger, thus obliterating or greatly reducing the flow through the lesion. This also provides a very narrow compressed sheath of vessels coming between the fingers that can be progressively clipped or coagulated and divided.

As so often happens when working in any one edge of the malformation, hemorrhage may become uncontrollable. If the surgeon finds that he is wasting time sucking and trying to see vessels without making any progress occluding them, he should pack the area and start down another area. If the same degree of hemorrhage occurs there, he should again pack and go back to the first which by this time may be reduced to the point where he can see the main bleeders, particularly just as the pack is removed. If this is not the case, he should repack the first area and start on a third area. It is extremely important that the surgeon does not panic and lose time simply sucking away at a bloody field without making any progress because the anesthetist is having trouble getting the blood pressure up. At that point, the surgeon should work all the more intensely as it may be his best chance to get some of the main bleeders. At this point, we never use hypotensives deliberately although we have, on occasions, convinced the anesthetists that it is advisable to withdraw 500 cc or so prior to starting and then have that ready to give back to the patient.

The fourth and final step must be the assurance that the lesion is completely removed. It is our belief that the postoperative disasters occur when parts of the fistula or a separate center are left behind without the surrounding supporting tissue that was there prior to the surgical intervention. It is here that intraoperative serial angiography is of inestimable value. Single films may be quite misleading. A series of six, taken at 1-second intervals, will assure the surgeon either that his removal is complete or else that there is a residual, and at that same time, it will show him exactly the location of any residual.

In summary, it should be emphasized that these lesions must be completely removed in order to assure against immediate or delayed postoperative bleeding. It should be remembered that removal of the lesion can only improve the circulation as it removes the low pressure steal. No nutrient function ever comes back out of the lesion but nutrient arteries may pass very close to the lesion. We suspect that when there are two or more major arteries contributing, there are probably two or more units of fistula. We have no proof of this in every instance, and we would be at great puzzlement to try to explain why there should be multiple angioblastic mistakes so closely adjacent to each other.

Cushing's admonition to all neurosurgery, although aimed at lesions now considered less formidable, was to the effect that the neurosurgeon could never relax his attention for one second because the "dice of the gods are loaded."

Vascular Malformations, edited by
R.R. Smith, A. Haerer and W.F. Russell.
Raven Press, New York © 1982.

Arteriovenous Malformations of the Posterior Cranial Fossa

Robert R. Smith and P. Shripathi Holla

*Department of Neurosurgery, University of Mississippi Medical Center,
Jackson, Mississippi 39216*

Although malformations of the posterior cranial fossa have been recognized since the mid-19th century, little progress in diagnostic methodology was made until the development of routine vertebral angiography only a few years ago. Both Cushing (2) and Dandy (4) recognized that, to be effective, the surgical approach required total obliteration of the communication. Both, however, also recognized the potential pitfalls of an operative attack and cautioned against operative treatment if other options were open. Poppen (10) warned that once removal of the malformation is started, it may be difficult if not impossible to retreat. The advice of these sage pioneers has been heeded and only within the past decade have these lesions attracted the attention of surgeons.

Little is actually known of the history of malformations of the posterior cranial fossa and there is no consensus as to best treatment. Matsumura et al. (7), who collected one of the largest series, 14 cases, were surprised that some of those initially considered to be inoperable could be resected. Viale et al. (14) pointed out that some of the malformations that appear to be within the brainstem actually lie on the surface and the telangiectatic lesion of the pons itself is comparatively rare. As posterior fossa angiography became more commonly employed, however, a distinct clinical pattern emerged. Nearly one-half of the patients presenting with subarachnoid hemorrhage will have some localizing signs. Sudden, nonlocalizing subarachnoid hemorrhage is also by far the most common clinical presentation (9). The lesion seems to imitate other neurological conditions, such as multiple sclerosis and trigeminal neuralgia in nonhemorrhagic cases. The patient recognizes a bruit in cases of dural arteriovenous malformations (AVM), and in AVMs of the posterior fossa a bruit is audible to the examiner in about one-third of all cases (5). Hydrocephalus of a slowly progressive type is present in a number of cases.

In light of recent developments in the therapy of AVMs in general, such as microsurgical excision, feeder artery ligation, and pellet embolization, it appears worthwhile to review a recent series of these cases. In defining AVMs, we have excluded all vascular tumors such as hemangioblastomas and vascular meningiomas, and likewise have not included those malformations having a predominant supratentorial location, such as the vein of Galen malformation. Dural malformations, located almost exclusively in the posterior cranial fossa, and receiving major blood supply from the posterior circulation, were included in this report.

METHODS

The case records of all patients admitted to the University of Mississippi Medical Center between the year 1965 and 1980 with a diagnosis of an AVM were reviewed. Cases admitted to the Jackson VA Center were also included if the malformation was located in the posterior cranial fossa. Radiographic materials, when relevant and available, were also reviewed. In all but two cases, recent followup data was obtained either by chart review, clinic visit, or by telephone consultation.

RESULTS

During the 15-year interval, vascular malformations of the posterior cranial fossa were identified in 14 patients.

The average age at which symptoms were noted was 39 years. The youngest patient in this series was 5 years of age and the oldest was 62 years. Most patients presented within the fourth decade. Approximately half were female, and 60% presented with acute subarachnoid hemorrhage. Four of the patients indicated a history of strenuous work at the time of subarachnoid hemorrhage, whereas two were engaged in light or less strenuous activity. Of those who presented with the clinical signs related to subarachnoid hemorrhage, acute headache and nausea and vomiting were described by all. In one-half of the cases the subarachnoid hemorrhage was nonlocalizing. Hydrocephalus and trigeminal neuralgia were encountered three times and once, respectively.

There was nothing typical of headaches in patients harboring AVMs who did not suffer from subarachnoid hemorrhage. Patients who noticed a pulse synchronous bruit were found ultimately to have dural AVMs. These were all the patients who complained of tinnitus. One patient who carried a diagnosis of multiple sclerosis presented with hearing loss in the right ear, sensory impairment on the right side of the face, a slight right hemiparesis, and ataxia. Another young patient presented with a slowly progressive right arm and leg weakness. On examination he was found to have a third nerve palsy, right hemiparesis and involvement of the left ninth, tenth, eleventh, and twelfth nerves (Tables 1 and 2).

TABLE 1. *Presenting symptoms*

Symptoms	No. of patients
Headache, nausea, and vomiting	9/14
Confusion to coma	4/14
Tinnitus	2/14
Diplopia	2/14
Slurred speech	2/14
Ataxia	2/14
Syncope	1/14
Vertigo	1/14
Backache	1/14

TABLE 2. *Presenting signs*

Signs	No. of patients
Nuchal rigidity	9/14
Brainstem signs (chronic)	4/14
Lower cranial nerve involvement	3/14
Bruit	3/14
Hemiparesis	2/14
Cerebellar signs	2/14
Dysarthria	2/14

All patients had lumbar punctures either preceding their hospitalization or shortly thereafter. In no case was there documented deterioration in neurological status or recurrent hemorrhage associated with puncture. All underwent routine cranial radiographic studies and angiography. In recent years, 3 patients had CT scans. Except in one case, plain radiographs of the skull were interpreted to be normal. Angiography, however, was positive in all cases (Figs. 1, 2, and 3B). Computerized tomographic scans were positive in 100% of the cases in which the examination was done (Figs. 3A and 4).

Two patients died from recurrent bleeding during the follow-up period. Of those who bled, 25% bled again within 3.3 years. Follow-up intervals varied from 1 year to 21 years. In 4 patients, the lesion was excised *in toto*, and in 5 conservative therapy was instituted. Embolization was accomplished in 2 patients, and 3 had shunting procedures because of hydrocephalus. In 2 patients, incomplete excision or feeder ligation was performed (Table 3).

In every case, AVM was supplied by multiple feeding vessels. In over 90% of the cases these were restricted to the posterior circulation including the posterior cerebral arteries. In every case, however, the predominant nutrient vessel could be identified. This served a useful purpose in classification of the malformation (Fig. 5). The most common predominant vessels supplying malformations of the posterior cranial fossa in this series were the superior cerebellar artery and the posterior inferior cerebellar artery. Venous drainage occurred predominantly through the lateral and sigmoid sinuses, rather than directly via the straight sinus (Fig. 6). In

TABLE 3. *Treatment*

Type of treatment	No. of patients
Surgery	
Excision	4/14
Ligation of the feeder	2/14
Shunt	3/14
Embolization	2/14
Conservative	5/14

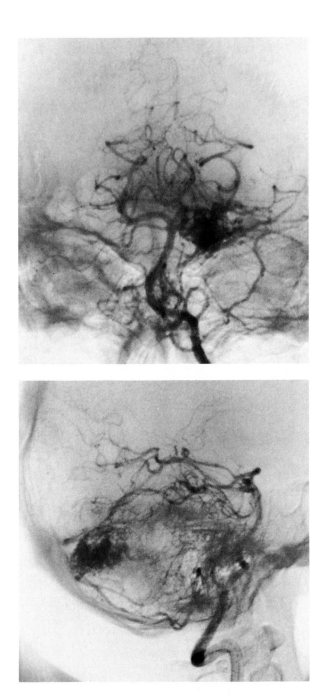

FIG. 1 (top and bottom). Arteriovenous malformation supplied predominantly by the inferior and superior cerebellar arteries.

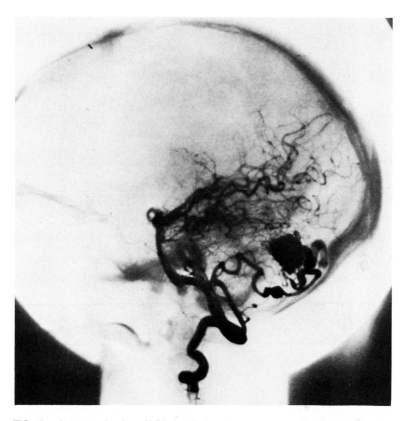

FIG. 2. An example of an AVM supplied by the posterior inferior cerebral artery.

addition to a large malformation served by multiple nutrient vessels, one case was complicated by the existence of two large intracranial aneurysms on major nutrient vessels.

DISCUSSION

Presumably, AVMs of the posterior cranial fossa are like their supratentorial counterparts and arise predominantly from prenatal factors. Between the 20 and 80-mm stage of development of the brain, segmental arteries and veins cross each other, and at this stage only a double layer of endothelial cells separates the primitive artery from the primitive vein. It is at this stage that breakdown of the endothelial wall occurs and communications develop. With development of the cerebellar hemispheres, the primitive artery–vein communication may be displaced a considerable distance from its origin but the primitive arterial channel and draining veins are usually well preserved. The primitive metencephalon receives its blood supply from

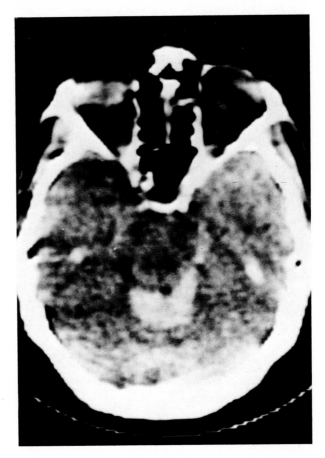

FIG. 3. A: A 50-year-old man presented with sudden occipital headache and nuchal rigidity. This CT scan indicates hematoma in the vermis dissecting into the fourth ventricle and subarachnoid cistern.

the superior cerebellar artery and drains through the ventral and dorsal myelencephalic vein. Ordinarily, during development, with reduced flow in these veins, they degenerate. However, with arterialized blood coursing through them, they persist and may be seen even in the adult with AVM of the posterior cranial fossa. In myelencephalic AVMs the anterior inferior cerebellar artery drains into a persistent myelencephalic vein which passes laterally and upwards into the transverse sinus (12). The arterial and venous components of dural malformations of the posterior cranial fossa are less well understood. Vidyasagar (13) presents convincing evidence that

FIG. 3B (top and bottom). The angiogram disclosed an AVM supplied by the vermian branches of the superior cerebellar artery.

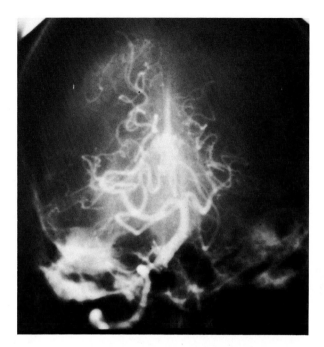

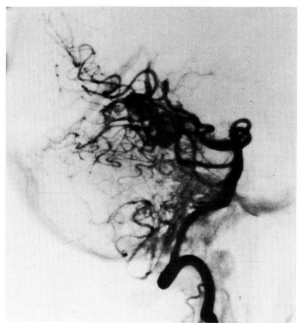

FIG. 3.

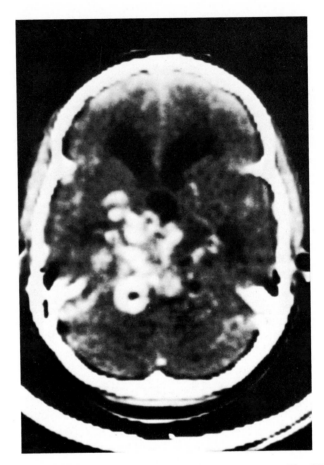

FIG. 4. A 32-year-old female carried a diagnosis of multiple sclerosis. The CT findings are typical of a vascular malformation with associated hydrocephalus (with contrast).

the meningeal artery, the internal carotid artery, the ophthalmic artery, and the occipital artery all may participate and even the vertebral artery may send a branch into the malformation. A prominent occipital artery is usually, but not necessarily, the primary feeder. Persistent embryonic veins drain the dural malformation into nearby lateral and sigmoid sinuses.

As McCormick et al. (8) have emphasized, virtually every type of malformation described in the supratentorial compartment may also be found in the posterior cranial fossa. Those who have gone to painstaking efforts to subclassify these malformations have brought out interesting features in the various vascular lesions. The telangiectatic lesions are found four to five times more often in the pons than

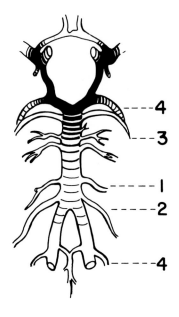

FIG. 5. Schematic diagram of the posterior circulation and the distribution of AVMs based on primary efferent feeding vessel.

in the cerebellar hemisphere (8). The arteriovenous type and the large venous types prefer the cerebellum over the brainstem two to one. It is well known that the AV type anomaly is by far more often associated with hemorrhage than the other groups (8). Of those in the posterior cranial fossa which have bled, at least 80% have both large arterial and venous channels (8). The most innocuous type of angioma appears to be the telangiectatic lesion, which is rarely associated with hemorrhage (8).

The so-called dural malformation, although usually supplied by both extracranial and intracranial nutrient vessels, should probably be considered separately. It carries a remarkably benign course with the loud bruit being the most common symptom that leads the patient to the physician. Apparently, the lesion hemorrhages infrequently (11). Unless the noise of the shunt produces annoying symptoms interfering with sleep or productivity, little therapy is indicated. The lesion may be obliterated surgically, but total excision of the malformation including the affected sinus must be undertaken. In one of our cases, there was relief of symptoms following pellet embolization. In another case, nutrient artery ligation was associated with the development of sensory changes in the face, suggestive of lateral medullary ischemia. Apparently, the vertebral artery steal increased after external carotid scalp vessels were ligated. Therefore, nutrient vessel ligation is not recommended in the management of these lesions.

Although hemorrhage was by far the most common presenting complaint, a small number of patients were admitted with a history of progressive neurological deficit somewhat suggestive of multiple sclerosis. The intermittent progressive-remission findings may have been associated with ischemia or hemorrhage. On clinical evidence

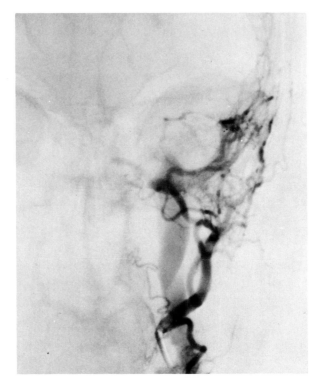

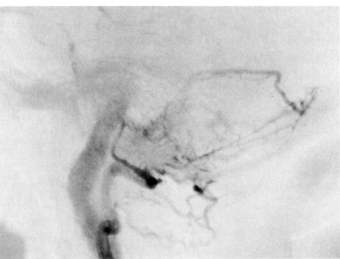

FIG. 6 (top and bottom). A 60-year-old female presented with tinnitus in the left ear and was found to have a pulse synchronous bruit over the left mastoid process. The dural malformation in this case was supplied by the external carotid artery and muscular branches of the vertebral artery, and drained into sigmoid sinus.

it was possible to localize these lesions to the mesencephalon. In one of our cases a good history of trigeminal neuralgia prompted the patient to seek attention. Fortunately, many of the patients who present with facial pain are unusually young and do have objective neurological signs that bring the question of a structural lesion to mind. In some, an audible bruit will help make the diagnosis but the exclusion of a brainstem glioma may be more difficult on clinical grounds. The unusually long period of progression is a distinctive feature.

Hydrocephalus associated with AVMs of the posterior cranial fossa may be of several types. In our series, both cases were presumed to be of the obstructive type and the patient's symptoms were partly relieved by a shunting procedure. Others, however, have noted difficulty in explaining the ventricular dilatation seen in some patients with malformations (8). There may be obvious brain atrophy associated with the stealing of blood. In other patients, however, there is a normal cortical pattern on CT scanning. We are led to wonder if arterial pressure in the great venous sinuses might interfere with absorption of cerebrospinal fluid from the Pacchionian granulations in some cases. If this is true, shunting might provide little relief. The hydrocephalus associated with AVMs is known to occur even in the absence of a prior history of subarachnoid hemorrhage.

In our series, posterior fossa AVMs constituted 15% of our total series, higher than in many series. One patient also had multiple aneurysms on the major nutrient artery of the malformation. Polycystic renal disease was encountered in another case. Otherwise, there was no history to suggest possible congenital factors in the development. There was an unusually high mortaility rate (14.5%) and this has also been noted by others (6,9). Perhaps this is related to the limited available space in the posterior fossa as well as to the proximity of such vital structures as the respiratory center. As with other vascular anomalies, activity may play some role in the cause of the initial hemorrhage with posterior fossa AVMs. Lusins (6) has reported hemorrhage from posterior fossa AVM after head injury. Hemorrhage followed a Valsalva maneuver in one of our cases and in others increased venous pressures seemed to precipitate the event.

In regard to therapy, certainly in those patients with dural malformations, unless the lesion is producing debilitating clinical signs, nonoperative therapy is warranted. Pellet, and perhaps even liquid, embolic agents may find a place in the treatment of this malformation. Feeder artery ligation is contraindicated and unless total excision can be carried out safely, it is probably wise to leave the malformation untreated. Occasionally, a dural malformation of the supratentorial space will undergo spontaneous remission and presumably this is true for those in the posterior cranial fossa (1). We have observed a waxing and waning course in several patients in our series who were treated nonoperatively.

Embolization, a therapeutic adjuvant in supratentorial AVMs, must play a less effective role in those of the posterior cranial fossa. Because of the straight position of the basilar artery in relation to its tributaries embolization is not practical in most cases. In each of the cases embolized with pellets there was unsatisfactory placement, although no serious complications were associated with their use. As suggested by Viale et al. (14), Matsumura et al. (7), and Chou et al. (3), many malformations that appear to penetrate the brainstem lie on its surface and these lesions may be excised *in toto*. By far the majority of those located in the cerebellar hemispheres can be excised and there has been little deficit associated with the procedure. We believe that the standard approach of occluding arterial nutrient vessels before disturbing the venous drainage is a good one for the posterior fossa lesion as well. This usually means circumferentially occluding nutrient arteries to the malformation before severing its attachment to the lateral or sigmoid sinus. In contrast to the approach recommended by Matsumura et al. (7) for lesions of the anterior aspect of the cerebellum, we prefer a bilateral supracerebellar approach when this is feasible. This provides excellent exposure of the malformation itself and the superior cerebellar arteries, the predominant supply of the superior cerebellar lesion. The transtentorial approach provides little access to either the arterial supply or venous drainage. Conservative management is still applicable to those malformations which seem to penetrate the brainstem, and those treated conservatively in our series have done well.

REFERENCES

1. Bitoh, S., and Sakaki, S. (1979): Spontaneous cure of dural arteriovenous malformation in the posterior fossa. *Surg. Neurol.*, 12:111–114.
2. Cushing, H., and Bailey, P. (1928): *Tumors Arising from the Blood Vessels of the Brain: Angiomatous Malformations and Hemangioblastomas*. pp. 219. Charles C Thomas, Springfield, Illinois.
3. Chou, N. S., Erickson, L. D., and Ortiz-Suarez, H. J. (1975): Surgical treatment of vascular lesions in the brainstem. *J. Neurosurg.*, 42:23–31.
4. Dandy, W. E. (1928): Arteriovenous aneurysms of the brain. *Arch. Surg.*, 17:190–243.
5. Logue, V., and Monckton, G. (1954): Posterior fossa angiomas. *Brain*, 77:252–273.
6. Lusins, J., and Sencer, W. (1976): Posterior fossa vascular malformation—Long term followup. *N. Y. State J. Med.*, 76:416–420.
7. Matsumura, H., Makita, Y., Someda, K., and Kondo, A. (1977): Arteriovenous malformations in the posterior fossa. *J. Neurosurg.*, 47:50–56.
8. McCormick, W. F., Hardman, J. M., and Boulter, T. R. (1968): Vascular malformations ("angiomas") of the brain, with special reference to those occurring in the posterior fossa. *J. Neurosurg.*, 20:241–251.
9. Perret, G., and Nishioka, H. (1966): Report of the cooperative study of intracranial aneurysms and subarachnoid hemorrhage, Section VI. Arteriovenous malformations. *J. Neurosurg.*, 25:467–490.
10. Poppen, J. L. (1968): Vascular surgery of the posterior fossa. *Clin. Neurosurg.*, 6:198–210.
11. Solis, O. J., Davis, K. R., and Ellis, G. T. (1977): Dural arteriovenous malformation associated with subdural and intracerebral hematoma: A CT scan and angiographic correlation. *Comput. Tomography*, 1:145–150.
12. Vidyasagar, C. (1979): Persistent embryonic veins in arteriovenous malformations of the posterior fossa. *Acta Neurochir.*, 48:67–82.
13. Vidyasagar, C. (1979): Persistent embryonic veins in arteriovenous malformations of the dura. *Acta Neurochir.*, 48:199–216.
14. Viale, G. L., Pau, A., and Viale, E. S. (1979): Surgical treatment of arteriovenous malformations of the posterior fossa. *Surg. Neurol.*, 12:379–384.

Vascular Malformations, edited by
R.R. Smith, A. Haerer and W.F. Russell.
Raven Press, New York © 1982.

Surgical Treatment of Large Cerebral Arteriovenous Malformations

Ghaus M. Malik

*Department of Neurological Surgery and Neurology, Henry Ford Hospital,
Detroit, Michigan 48202*

Although in the last half century there has been a tremendous change in the treatment of arteriovenous malformations (AVM), problems still exist in the management of deeply located and very large malformations. It is now well established that the only ideal treatment is total excision of the lesion (15). Several recent large series attest to the fact that surgical excision in the majority of cases can be done with reasonable mortality and morbidity (4,14,17,21). The results are certainly better than the natural history reported by Michelsen (11). He estimated that the long-term mortality is approximately 18%, and morbidity leading to disability occurs in 30% of patients. Troupp et al. (22) reported similar results in 137 patients followed for over 21 years. Only 40 patients were reported well, 30 were considered to be in fair condition, 40 were disabled, and 21 had died (14 as a result of AVM and 7 from other causes).

There has been a tendency to a less aggressive treatment of the large malformations, citing technical problems in their removal because of the size and large shunt. Some of these have been partially treated with embolization (9), and others with combined embolization and surgical excision (5,6,20). As late as 1979, Drake (4) stated that it was not a question of whether large AVMs can be removed with very low mortality; it was whether they should be, in the face of a very real possibility of a devastating defect. He divided the arteriovenous malformations into small (<2.5 cm), moderate (2.5–5.0 cm) and large (>5.0 cm), whereas others have defined large malformations differently. Parkinson and Bachers (14) and Raskind and Weiss (16) regard lesions >2.0 cm as large, whereas Sang and Wilson (17) regard AVMs of > 4.0 cm in size as large.

This report is based on personal experience with surgical excision of large AVMs (>5 cm) in 8 patients without any adjunctive therapy such as preoperative or intraoperative embolization. At the time of surgery, these patients ranged from 16 to 54 years of age. One-half had arterial supply from all three major cerebral vessels (anterior, middle, and posterior cerebral arteries); in the other 4 cases, two of these major vessels contributed to the malformation. All 6 patients who had contribution from the ipsilateral anterior cerebral artery had the filling of this vessel primarily on contralateral carotid injection, suggesting that a "steal phenomenon" existed. This pattern was normalized after removal of the malformation. In addition, there was distinct supply from meningeal branches of the occipital artery and tentorial vessels in at least one patient. In all cases, there was drainage into both the superficial and deep venous systems. Our operative approach is described in some detail.

Preoperative Evaluation

Detailed selective four-vessel angiography is the most vital component of pre-operative evaluation. Computerized axial tomography, with transverse and coronal views, has added significant information regarding the extent of the malformation and its relationship to the ventricular system. The angiograms should be reviewed with great care to check for associated aneurysms, particularly on the main feeding artery. If there is an aneurysm present along with the malformation, the former needs treatment prior to the excision of the malformation because the aneurysm is likely to bleed once the arterial supply to the malformation has been interrupted because of higher pressure in the parent vessel.

A majority of the patients are in a young age group and are good risk patients. In older patients, complete medical evaluation is a necessity. Recently we have started to obtain neuropsychological evaluation as a baseline for later postoperative follow-up. Preliminary results indicate that the deficits noted in very large malformations not only point to brain dysfunction in the area of the malformation, but show rather widespread involvement of both hemispheres. Depending on the extent of the lesion, the patient is typed and cross-matched for several units of blood, and the blood bank is alerted to the possibility of the need for more blood in the operating room.

Operative Procedure

An arterial line and at least two large intravenous lines are established. A Foley catheter is also inserted to monitor urinary output and, if necessary, to permit the use of osmotic diuretics (mannitol). This has not been necessary in the cases to be reported here.

Every effort is made to position the patient without much distortion of the head in order to maintain good orientation. A generous craniotomy is fashioned, making several burr holes and preferably using the Gigli saw, rather than craniotome, to avoid injury to the dura, because some of the malformations receive blood supply from the meningeal vessels and the dura is quite vascular. The malformation itself may be adherent to the dura, and undue traction might start premature bleeding. A large craniotomy helps identify the draining veins and even some feeding vessels, and if brain swelling should occur, there is more room to accommodate the swollen brain. For a parasagittal exposure, the craniotomy is extended exactly to the midline. The dura is opened with great care, keeping in mind the orientation of venous drainage and the possibility of the AVM being adherent to the dura. Should an opening be made in a large venous channel, this is closed with a small muscle or Gelfoam[1] stamp sutured to the dura. Although some surgeons advocate ligating one

---

[1]The Upjohn Company, Kalamazoo, Michigan.

draining vein and using this as a guide to isolate the malformation, it is important to spare the venous drainage as long as possible. Our preference is to isolate and ligate the feeding arteries and maintain the veins until the malformation has been well isolated. If there is a large surface presentation, as in Case VII (Fig. 7C), cortical incision is made very close to the obvious malformation. None of the vessels farther away from the malformation, such as major branches of the middle cerebral artery, are ligated. Most convexity malformations of any size are roughly cone shaped, with the base at the surface and the apex at the ventricular wall. The malformations have a plane of cleavage below the cortex, a pseudocapsule of gliotic brain. Every effort is made to find this area of gliosis early and it is followed throughout. The feeding vessels are ligated as they approach the lesion, and dissection is continued along the malformation. The smaller arterial feeders are coagulated and divided, while the larger feeding vessels are occluded with "U" Hemoclips[2] as well as cauterized before they are divided. In cases where surface presentation is only limited to emerging arterialized veins, as in Case IV (Fig. 4), one would have to start with a smaller cortical incision until the malformation is approached, and this might have to be adjusted, depending on the extent of the lesion.

Surgical loupes are used whenever magnification is desired. The coagulation and interruption of arterial feeders is generally accomplished with monopolar coagulation; however, thin enlarged vessels in the white matter, at times, require bipolar coagulation. These vessels should be grasped and coagulated with care; otherwise they may be torn more proximally and have to be followed back into the brain tissue to be secured with difficulty. In the posterior lesions, the deep feeding vessels arising from the posterior cerebral artery pose some difficulty in ligation. Should bleeding start from a loop of the malformation, it could be controlled with coagulation if the bleeding point is quite obvious, or stopped with gentle pressure with a brain retractor or a cottonoid. This area should be left alone for a while and dissection started at another point. One must be careful not to wander away into the adjacent brain. On the other hand, leaving any loops of the malformation outside the line of dissection should also be avoided, because this could certainly cause bleeding and swelling of the brain.

As most of these malformations extend to the lateral ventricle and drain into the internal venous system, great care is taken as the ependyma is reached. The subependymal veins are isolated, coagulated, and divided. This becomes simpler if all the arterial component has been eliminated and, particularly if a superficial draining vein is left intact. In a malformation involving the ventricle itself, there is involvement of the choroid plexus. All abnormal vessels need to be coagulated and excised.

Deliberate hypotension was not used in these cases. It is our belief that, with large malformations, there is a high potential of causing ischemia of the normal brain, since relatively increased blood flow will continue through the large arterio-

[2]Edward Weck & Company, Inc., Long Island City, New York.

venous fistula, even at a lower pressure. The head of the table is kept slightly elevated to avoid brain congestion and to facilitate venous drainage.

Postoperative Care

The patients are followed very closely for the possibility of postoperative hemorrhage. Urgent surgical intervention is necessary if postoperative hemorrhage should occur, since this is arterial in nature and would lead to herniation very quickly. Dexamethasone is used intraoperatively and continued for a few days postoperatively. Postoperative angiography, to confirm complete excision of the malformation, is essential. If any residual malformation is found, it should be excised promptly. It was shown by Amacher et al. (1) that even a tiny portion of an AVM left behind is dangerous in that it could enlarge and bleed again; 6 of the 14 known incomplete resections of their series rebled. The only patient in this series having a residual malformation, even though extremely small, bled 6 months postoperatively.

CASE REPORTS

Case I: J. M., a 44-year-old right-handed white male, presented with generalized seizures. Neurologically the patient was intact. Computed axial tomography showed a large lesion in the left frontal area consistent with the AVM. Cerebral angiography confirmed the presence of an extensive AVM being supplied by the branches of middle and anterior cerebral arteries (Fig. 1A). There was also filling of the anterior cerebral artery from the contralateral side (Fig. 1B). At surgery, the malformation

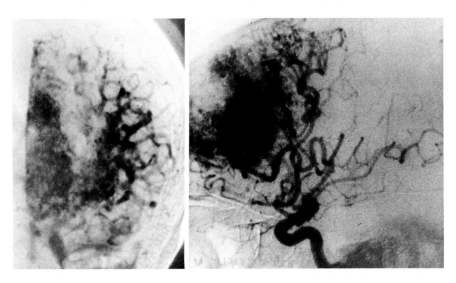

FIG. 1.A: Left carotid angiogram (AP and lateral views) showing the extent of the malformation filling from branches of the middle and anterior cerebral arteries.

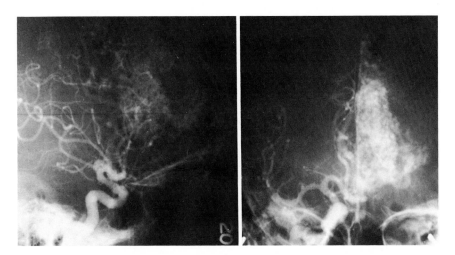

FIG. 1.B: Right carotid angiogram (AP and lateral views). Note visualization of the malformation through its supply from the left anterior cerebral artery filled from the contralateral side.

occupied most of the frontal lobe (Fig. 1C) and was excised without any deterioration of the patient's neurological function or other postoperative problems. Postoperative angiography (Fig. 1D) confirmed total excision of the malformation with preservation of normal vessels.

Case II: R. K., a 19-year-old right-handed white male had two episodes of subarachnoid hemorrhage at age 16 and was diagnosed as having a large malformation in the left parietal region. Surgical excision was recommended but was refused by the family. Three years later he had another subarachnoid hemorrhage, but suffered no deficit. Angiography again showed the malformation being supplied by the middle cerebral artery (Fig. 2A), the posterior cerebral artery (Fig. 2B) and the anterior cerebral artery filling from the contralateral side. Excision of the malformation was accomplished without any complications or neurological deficit, and postoperative angiograms showed complete removal of the malformation (Fig. 2C).

Case III: C. S., a 16-year-old right-handed white female, was found, during workup for intractable headaches, to have a large left occipital AVM. The malformation was supplied by the branches of the middle (Fig. 3A) and posterior cerebral (Fig. 3B) arteries with major drainage into the great vein of Galen and the straight sinus (Fig. 3C). The malformation was removed completely, as confirmed by angiography (Figs. 3D and E). Except for an expected right hemonymous field defect, she has had no other problems and remains free of headaches.

Case IV: J. P., a 29-year-old right-handed white female, had suffered from severe headaches and one episode of brief visual impairment. This led to the diagnosis of a large right frontal AVM supplied by the anterior and middle cerebral arteries.

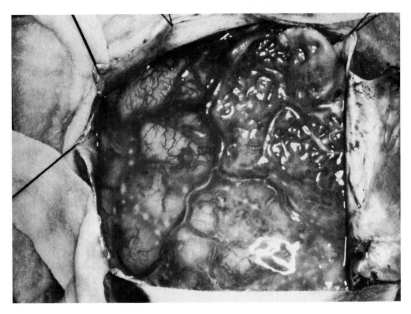

FIG. 1.C: Surface presentation of the malformation. Dura has been reflected to the midline.

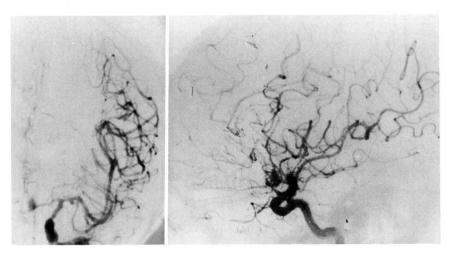

FIG. 1.D: Postoperative left carotid angiogram showing total excision of the AVM and preservation of normal vessels.

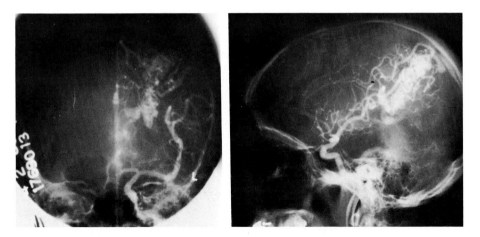

FIG. 2.A: Left carotid angiogram (AP and lateral views) showing supply from the middle cerebral artery.

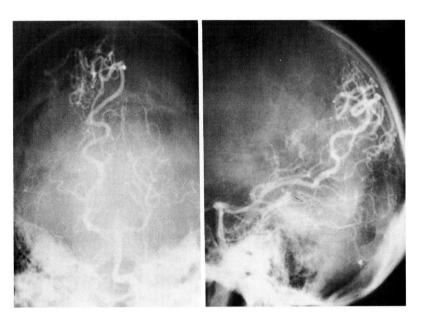

FIG. 2.B: Vertebral angiogram (AP and lateral views) showing supply from the posterior cerebral artery. (Anterior cerebral artery also contributed to the malformation and filled on the right carotid angiogram).

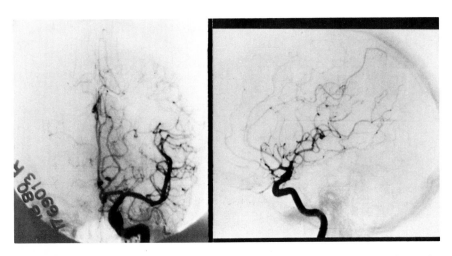

FIG. 2.C: Postoperative left carotid angiogram (AP and lateral views). Supply from other vessels also confirmed to have been eliminated.

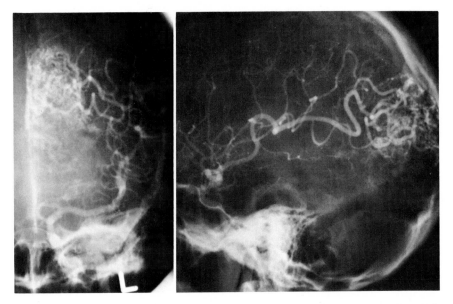

FIG. 3.A: Left carotid angiogram (AP and lateral views) showing supply from the middle cerebral artery.

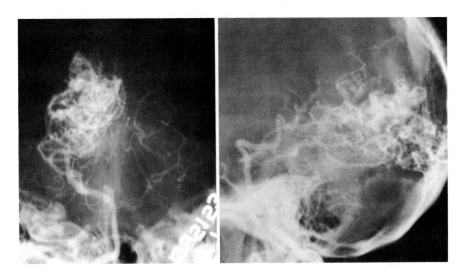

FIG. 3.B: Vertebral angiogram (AP and lateral views) indicating contribution from the posterior cerebral artery.

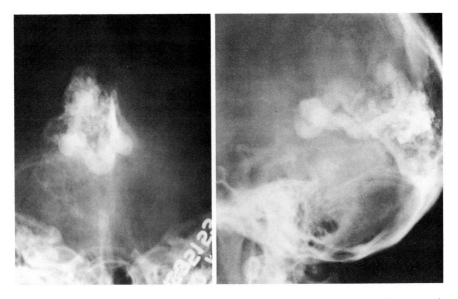

FIG. 3.C: Venous phase (AP and lateral views) showing primary drainage into the great vein of Galen and straight sinus.

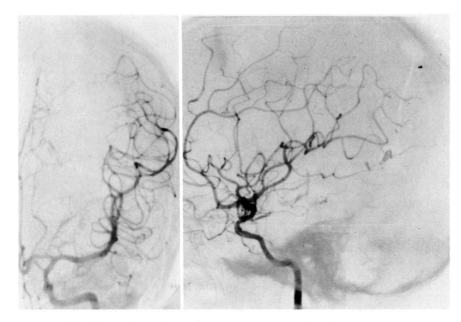

FIG. 3.D: Left carotid angiogram, postoperative (AP and lateral views).

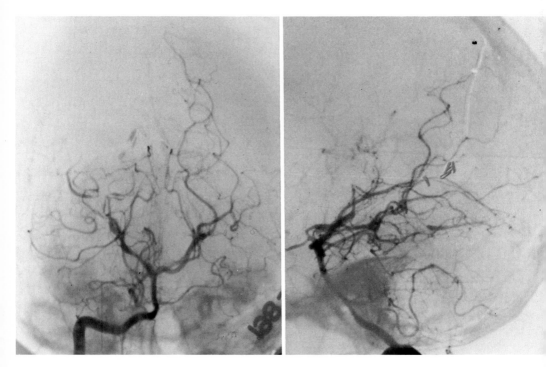

FIG. 3.E: Vertebral angiogram, postoperative (AP and lateral views).

Except for two large draining veins, very little of the malformation presented on the surface (Fig. 4). Removal of the malformation was difficult, mainly due to inadequate initial exposure and not staying completely outside of the malformation. The operation took 16 hours to complete, and the patient required 23 units of blood. However, she had a normal postoperative course and experienced no deficits. Postoperative angiograms showed total excision of the malformation.

Case V: J. M., a 29-year-old right-handed white male, started having generalized seizures 5 years prior to his operation in 1979. These seizures were poorly controlled with Dilantin and phenobarbital. In addition, he had multiple episodes of subarachnoid hemorrhage. He was diagnosed as having a large right parietal AVM; however, he was told that the malformation was too large to be considered for surgery. The patient presented to us with another subarachnoid hemorrhage. The malformation received its blood supply from the middle cerebral artery (Fig. 5A), the posterior cerebral artery (Fig. 5B) and the anterior cerebral artery filling from the opposite side (Fig. 5C). Because of the proximity of sensory motor cortex, the initial cortical incision was made extremely close to the malformation and, in the deeper dissection, part of the malformation was left outside the line of resection. This produced extra bleeding and swelling of the adjacent brain. The patient developed left homonymous hemianopsia and moderate left hemiparesis. On the postoperative angiogram, one small abnormal vessel was seen (Fig. 5D). It was suspected that he had a small residual malformation, but, in view of his deficit, surgery was

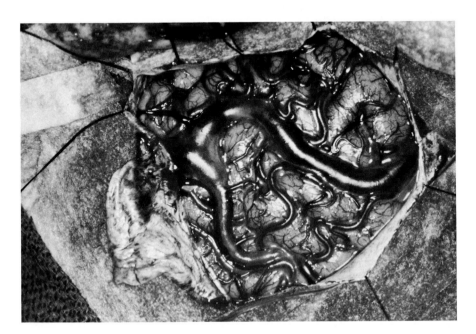

FIG. 4. Operative photograph only shows two large draining veins but no surface presentation was noted. Dura has been reflected to the midline.

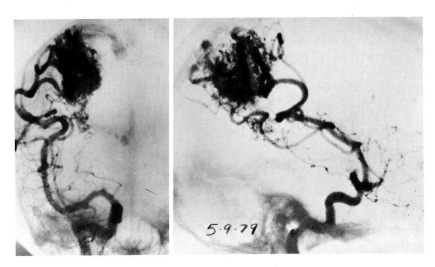

FIG. 5.A: AP and lateral views of the right carotid angiogram showing the middle cerebral artery supply to the malformation.

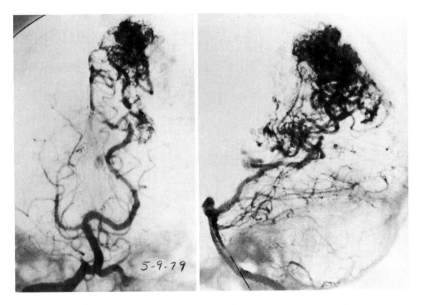

FIG. 5.B: Vertebral angiogram (AP and lateral views) indicating supply from the posterior cerebral artery.

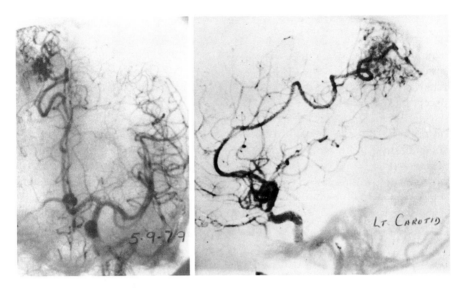

FIG. 5.C: Left carotid angiogram (AP and lateral views) showing supply from the right anterior cerebral artery filled from the opposite side.

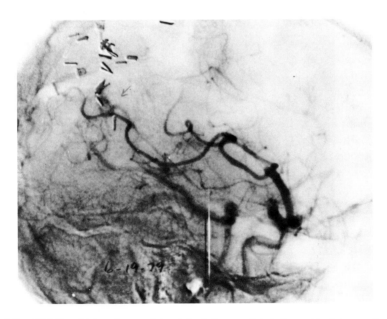

FIG. 5.D: Right brachial angiogram (lateral view). Arrow points to the residual abnormal vessel.

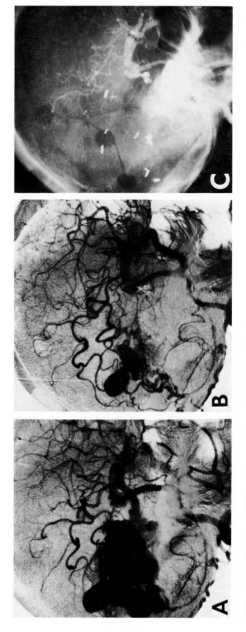

FIG. 6.A: Right brachial angiogram (lateral view) showing large malformation. Note extremely large size of posterior cerebral artery. **B:** Right brachial angiogram (lateral view) shows clipping of the posterior cerebral artery. Note better visualization of middle cerebral supply as well as the meningeal vessel from the occipital artery and tentorium. **C:** Right brachial angiogram (lateral view) shows complete excision of the malformation.

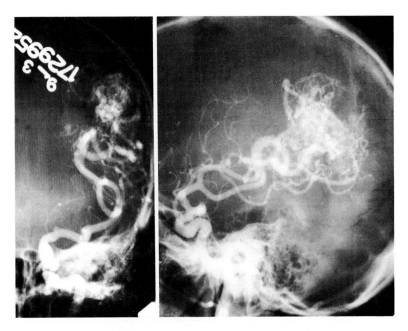

FIG. 7.A: Left carotid angiogram (AP and lateral views) shows the middle cerebral artery supply.

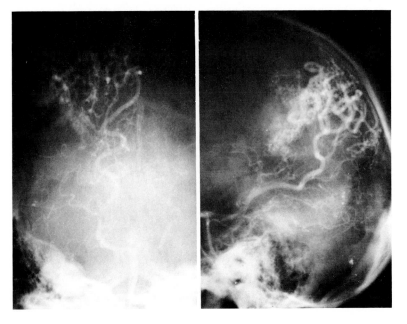

FIG. 7.B: Vertebral angiogram (AP and lateral) shows supply from the posterior cerebral artery.

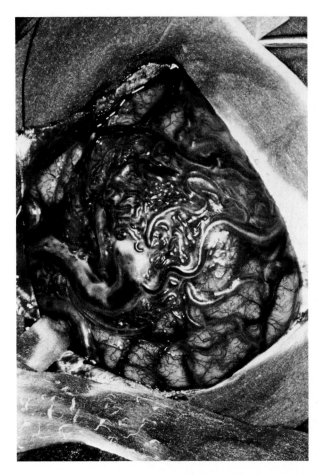

FIG. 7.C: Operative photograph showing large surface presentation. Note extremely large draining veins.

Postoperative angiograms confirmed complete excision of the malformation (Figs. 7D and E). Hemiparesis completely resolved, as did speech difficulty. She has been left with some difficulty in reading and calculations. The seizures were difficult to control for a time, but now her seizures are well controlled with medications.

Case VIII: S. G., a 33-year-old right-handed white female, presented with seizures. Studies revealed a large posterior temporal AVM supplied by the branches of middle and posterior cerebral arteries. The malformation was totally excised without any postoperative complications. She had minimal depression of the left upper quadrant visual field on both sides which completely resolved in 2 months. Total excision of the malformation was confirmed by postoperative angiography.

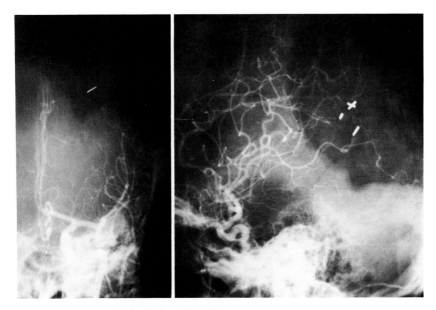

FIG. 7.D: Left carotid angiogram, postoperative (AP and lateral views), showing complete excision of the malformation.

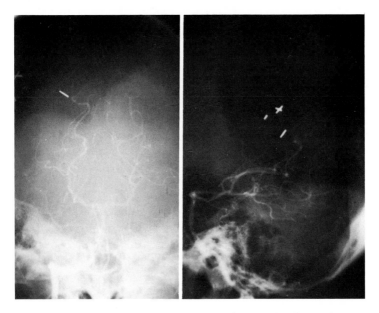

FIG. 7.E: Vertebral angiogram, postoperative (AP and lateral views), showing total excision of the malformation.

DISCUSSION

In the past few years there has been a tremendous proliferation of approaches to the treatment of AVMs of the brain. The now more conservative approach of the 1960s of resection after hemorrhage, intractable headache, or seizures for lesions away from the important areas of the brain, has given way to the surgical removal of the malformations in the motor strip, corpus callosum, and similar areas without producing significant deficits (2,8,24). Parkinson (13) and Stein (21) have found stereoangiography useful, a technique not available to many neurosurgeons. Embolization, popularized by Leussenhop et al. (9), has been refined further and, in addition to spheres, plastic materials and flexible and detachable balloon catheters have been advocated (3,18). Preoperative embolization has been used in selected cases by many (5,6,20), and intraoperative embolization has also been reported as an adjunct to definitive surgical excision (4). Walder (23) has found cryosurgical treatment, by freezing AVMs, to be ineffective. Finally, Kjellberg et al. (7) have advocated proton beam irradiation for deep inaccessible malformations which needs a longer period for evaluation of end results and, from the preliminary evidence, does not diminish a large lesion. None of these approaches has been proven to be favored over all others.

As is evident from the recent reports (4,14,17,21), small and moderate-sized malformations can be excised with reasonable mortality and morbidity. The larger malformations, however have received less aggressive treatment. Many large series only show a small number of large lesions. Drake (4) reported 13 cases out of 166 as being large; however, it is not clear as to how many of these were treated by surgical excision, since some of the cases were just explored or treated only with embolization. There were 7 cases with large malformations (>4.0 cm) in 31 cases reported by Sang and Wilson (17). Only 4 of these 7 were totally excised, whereas partial ligation of the feeding vessels was done in the other 3. There were 2 deaths in the group treated with total excision. Stein and Wolpert (21) have reported on their experience in 55 patients undergoing surgical resection, along with preoperative embolization; however, the authors did not define the size of the malformations included in their report.

Embolization as the sole treatment for these large malformations or as an adjunct to surgery has also been advocated (9,18,20). Theoretically, this seems to be attractive, particularly in the posteriorly located lesions with major supply from the posterior cerebral artery. In this volume, we have seen elegant demonstrations of catheterization, embolization, and balloon occlusion treatment of the cerebral vascular malformations; however, these approaches are not without problems or risks. Simple embolization may not treat the lesion completely and, therefore, does not prevent recurrent hemorrhage (10). Embolization certainly increases the number of procedures performed on the patient and the length of hospital stay, exposing the patient to further hazards. Fleisher and Tindall (5), in reporting on their experience with combined treatment (embolization and surgical excision) of 7 giant AVMs of the posterior cerebral hemisphere, stressed the point that preoperative embolization did not significantly alter the blood flow and, hence, potential of bleeding at the time of operation. In this series, one patient died from a gram-negative meningitis. The outcome in the remaining 6 patients, despite transient neurological deficit in 3 patients, was excellent.

In this report we have discussed the treatment of large AVMs fed by two or three major cerebral vessels. Our approach has been conventional, utilizing the equipment and technique available to most neurosurgeons. Monopolar coagulation has been quite adequate for hemostasis. Bipolar coagulation, however, might be needed in some instances for occlusion of enlarged thin vessels in the white matter. The use of an operating microscope has been advocated by some as most helpful (8,21,24); however, in giant malformations, where a larger perspective is always necessary and rapid control of bleeding is a constant problem, the necessity to reduce operative time in already long operations has made microscopic magnification a hindrance rather than an asset. Surgical loupes have been found to be adequate if some magnification is desired during the procedure.

Spetzler et al. (19), Drake (4), and Mullen et al. (12) have reported seeing tremendous cerebral edema and intracerebral hemorrhages in the large malformations after the blood supply from major vessels, particularly the middle cerebral artery, is suddenly occluded. These changes are believed to be related to diversion of an already increased blood flow to normal vessels which do not tolerate that pressure. In our cases, only one patient had transient swelling in the adjacent brain, and this was definitely related to losing the plane of cleavage and leaving some malformation behind. This was easily controlled as the remaining malformation was excised. At least in cases reported by Mullen et al. (12), there was sudden occlusion of the main middle cerebral artery which certainly would increase the pressure in normal vessels. The problem, although most likely real, should be much less frequent if the feeding vessels are coagulated individually exactly next to the malformation, and normal branches of the main artery are left intact.

I have not used intraoperative angiography advocated by some authors (14), as it seems quite cumbersome and the resolution necessary to check for tiny malformations would seem to be lacking. Instead, selective postoperative angiography is done early to confirm complete excision of the malformation. If residual AVM is noted, it should be removed promptly. Although I do not use routine prophylactic antibiotics, and none were used in these cases, it seems that since these procedures take a longer time and increase the risk of infection, prophylactic antibiotics may be valuable.

In conclusion, 8 cases of large cerebral AVMs, treated by direct surgical excision, are presented. Our results have proven very acceptable and, therefore, encourage me to emphasize that these large AVMs can be successfully removed with the approach as outlined.

ACKNOWLEDGMENTS

I am extremely grateful to James I. Ausman, M.D., Ph.D. Chairman, Department of Neurological Surgery and Neurology, and my other associates for their advice in the preparation of this manuscript. Special thanks to Sandra Marino for secretarial help and Medical Arts and Photography Department for the illustrations.

REFERENCES

1. Amacher, A. L., Allcock, J. M., and Drake, C. G. (1972): Cerebral angiomas: The sequelae of surgical treatment. *J. Neurosurg.*, 37:571–575.
2. Andreussi, L., Cama, A., Grossi, G., Marino, C., and Servato, R. (1979): Microsurgical excision of a strioinsular arteriovenous malformation. *Surg. Neurol.*, 12:499–502.
3. Debrun, G., Lacour, P., Caron, J., Hurth, M., Comoy, J., and Keravel, Y. (1978): Detachable balloon and caliberated-leak balloon techniques in the treatment of cerebral vascular lesions. *J. Neurosurg.*, 49:635–649.
4. Drake, C. G. (1979): Cerebral arteriovenous malformations: Considerations for and experience with surgical treatment in 166 cases. *Clin. Neurosurg.*, 26:145–208.
5. Fleisher, A. S., and Tindall, G. T. (1979): Giant arteriovenous malformations of the posterior cerebral hemisphere (abstract). *Neurosurgery*, 4:549–550.
6. Friedman, P., Salazar, J. L., and Sugar, O. (1978): Embolization and surgical excision of giant arteriovenous malformations. *Surg. Neurol.*, 9:149–152.
7. Kjellberg, R. N., Poletti, C. E., Robertson, G. H., and Adams, D. A. (1978): Bragg peak proton beam treatment of arteriovenous malformations of the brain (with emphasis on noninvasive methods of diagnosis and treatment). In: *Neurological Surgery*, edited by R. Carrea, pp. 181–187. Excerpta Medica, Amsterdam.
8. Kunc, Z. (1949): Surgery of arteriovenous malformations in the speech and motor sensory regions. *J. Neurosurg.*, 40:293–303.
9. Luessenhop, A. J., Kachmann, R., Shevlin, W., and Ferrero, A. A. (1965): Clinical evaluation of artificial embolization in the management of large cerebral arteriovenous malformations. *J. Neurosurg.*, 23:400–417.
10. Luessenhop, A. J., and Presper, J. M. (1975): Surgical embolization of cerebral arteriovenous malformations through internal carotid and vertebral arteries. *J. Neurosurg.*, 42:443–451.
11. Michelson, W. J. (1979): Natural history and pathophysiology of arteriovenous malformations. *Clin. Neurosurg.*, 26:307–313.
12. Mullen, S., Brown, F. D., and Patronas, N.J. (1979): Hyperemia and ischemia problems of surgical treatment of arteriovenous malformations. *J. Neurosurg.*, 51:757–764.
13. Parkinson, D. (1969): Rapid serial simultaneous biplane stereoscopic angiography: An aid in the surgical management of cerebral arteriovenous malformations. *Clin. Neurosurg.*, 16:179–184.
14. Parkinson, D., and Bachers, G. (1980): Arteriovenous malformations: Summary of 100 consecutive supratentorial cases. *J. Neurosurg.*, 53:285–299.
15. Pia, H. W., Gleave, J. R. W., Grote, E., and Zierski, J. Editors, (1975): Summary and conclusion. In: *Cerebral Angiomas—Advances in Diagnosis and Therapy*, pp. 279–281. Springer-Verlag, New York, Heidelberg, Berlin.
16. Raskind, R., and Weiss, S. R. (1971): Arteriovenous malformations: Follow-up in 68 cases. *Vasc. Surg.*, 5:30–35.
17. Sang, U. H., and Wilson, C. B. (1975): Surgical treatment of intracranial vascular malformations. *West. Med. J.*, 112:175–183.
18. Sano, K., Jimbo, M., Saito, I., and Basugi, N. (1975): Artificial embolization of inoperable angioma with polymerizing substance. In: *Cerebral Angiomas—Advances in Diagnosis and Therapy*, edited by H. W. Pia, J. R. W. Gleave, E. Grote, and J. Zierski, pp. 222–229. Springer-Verlag, New York, Heidelberg, Berlin.
19. Spetzler, R. F., Wilson, C. B., Weinstein, P., Mehdorn, M., Townsend, J., and Telles, D. (1978): Normal perfusion pressure breakthrough theory. *Clin. Neurosurg.*, 25:651–672.
20. Stein, B. M., and Wolpert, S. M. (1977): Surgical and emboli treatment of cerebral arteriovenous malformations. *Surg. Neurol.*, 7:359–369.
21. Stein, B. M., and Wolpert, S. M. (1980): Arteriovenous malformations of the brain. *Arch. Neurol.*, 37:69–75.
22. Troupp, H., Marttila, I., and Halonen, V. (1970): Arteriovenous malformations of the brain; prognosis without operation. *Acta Neurochir.*, 22:125–128.

23. Walder, H. A. D. (1975): Freezing arteriovenous anomalies in the brain, (cryosurgical treatment). In: *Cerebral Angiomas: Advances in Diagnosis and Therapy*, edited by H. W. Pia, J. R. W. Gleave, E. Grote, and J. Zierski, pp. 183–193. Springer-Verlag, New York, Heidelberg, Berlin.
24. Yasargil, M. G., Jain, K. K., Antic, J., and Laciga, R. (1976): Arteriovenous malformations of the splenium of the corpus callosum: Microsurgical treatment. *Surg. Neurol.*, 5:5–14.

Vascular Malformations, edited by
R. R. Smith, A. Haerer and W. F. Russell.
Raven Press, New York © 1982.

Pellet Embolization of Central Nervous System Arteriovenous Malformations

William F. Russell and Robert R. Smith

Departments of Radiology and Neurosurgery, University of Mississippi Medical Center, Jackson, Mississippi 39216

INTRODUCTION AND HISTORY

The natural history of arteriovenous malformations (AVM) of the brain results in a high incidence of morbidity and mortality, especially from the propensity to bleed. Surgical removal is the ideal treatment. This can be accomplished when the malformation is small and when it is not located in too vital an area of the brain to allow obliteration. The risk of surgery in large and less accessible lesions can be too great to intervene. Embolization as an alternative treatment in this group of patients was first conceived by Luessenhop in 1960 (5). His technique employed direct operative exposure and catheterization of the carotid arteries. In 1972 Kricheff and associates (4) refined the technique using a percutaneous transfemoral catheter approach, thereby eliminating needs for surgical incision and for general anesthesia. The current status of particulate embolization has recently been summarized by Stein and Wolpert (9). Berenstein and Kricheff (1) have discussed advantages and disadvantages of various embolic agents and catheter delivery systems.

Embolization has been performed at our institution since 1974.

MATERIALS AND METHODS

The femoral artery was catheterized with a Seldinger technique. Selective catheterization of the cerebral vessel to be embolized was accomplished in conventional fashion with a 5.0 French (Fr.) Hans Newton curved polyethelene catheter. A 260 cm 0.035 guide wire was then utilized to exchange catheters, leaving the guide in the selected vessel. A 100-cm polyethylene embolization catheter (O.D. 11.0 Fr.) was introduced with the aid of a 110 cm coaxial polyethylene catheter (O.D. 7.2 Fr.) over the guide wire and advanced to the desired level in the selected cerebral artery. This catheter and specially bored stopcock and adapter will allow passage of spheres up to 3.0 mm in diameter. Smaller catheters were used when the size of the AVM did not require emboli greater than 1.0 mm in diameter.

Radiopaque barium-impregnated silicone spheres were placed with small forceps singly or in groups of two or three into the hub of the saline filled stopcock. No air bubbles were allowed to enter the system when the saline filled syringe was connected. The sphere or spheres were flushed forward via hand injection when the stopcock was opened.

The patient was monitored clinically by the neurosurgeon in attendance throughout the procedure and examined after each injection. A plain radiograph was used to establish whether initial pellets lodged within the AVM. Preliminary, progress, and terminal arteriograms were performed employing uniform catheter placement and injector settings during each. Illustrative cases are described.

Case 1: This 58-year-old black male was presented to Jackson Veteran's Administration Hospital for evaluation of a seizure disorder. His illness began in early childhood when he first began to hear "roaring sounds" and smell "terrible odors." His problem initially was categorized as temporal lobe seizures, but for the past 17 years he has progressed to having grand mal seizures as well. Neurological examination was within normal limits. Computerized tomographic (CT) brain scan showed an enhancing cortical lesion in the right posterior temporal lobe. An arteriogram then revealed an arteriovenous malformation supplied almost entirely by a single enlarged posterior temporal branch of the right middle cerebral artery (Fig. 1). He was considered to be a candidate for embolization based on principles stated in Table 1 and on assessment of the surgical alternatives by the neurosurgeon. The procedure began with 1.5 mm spheres which were documented on AP and lateral radiographs to lodge within the AVM. Twenty-five of these were placed without

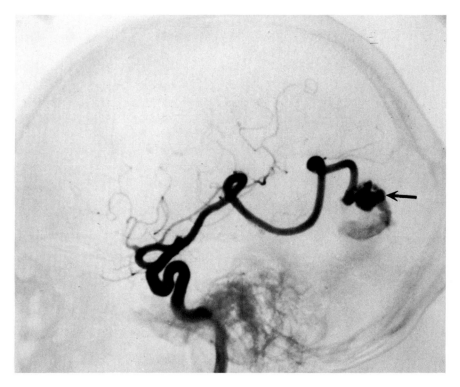

FIG. 1A. A small posterior parietal lobe AVM is supplied by a single enormously dilated middle cerebral arterial branch.

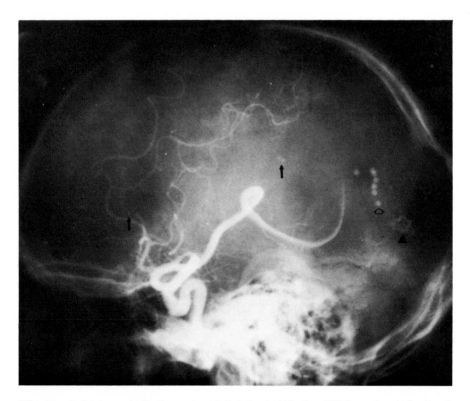

FIG. 1B. Following embolization, note pellets lodged within the AVM (*arrowhead*), lined up in the distal portion of the feeding artery (*open arrow*), and astray in normal branches (*arrows*). Anterior cerebral perfusion is improved.

neurological change. The arteriogram at this point revealed that 3 pellets had gone astray, occluding one frontal lobe branch (1 pellet) and one parietal lobe branch (2 pellets). The AVM still filled similarly to the original angiogram. Decision was made to continue. Eight pellets 25 mm in diameter were then introduced singly and fluoroscopic observation of test injections showed progressive decrease in flow through the AVM. Complete stasis of flow in the feeding branch was observed on the eighth pellet when the patient also experienced a sudden change in speech and nausea at that time. The procedure was ended. A final arteriogram was performed demonstrating total obliteration of the AVM as well as decreased perfusion of normal middle cerebral branches. The patient was somewhat disoriented and had left-sided weakness immediately following the procedure, but his hand grip was back to normal the next day, and he was more alert. He was discharged one week later with no clinically detectable deficit. A CT scan prior to discharge showed no evidence of infarction. The stray pellets, as well as the pellets within the AVM, were well demonstrated.

Case 2: This 50-year-old white male had chronic headaches for 20 years before he developed a subarachnoid hemorrhage in 1973. Workup at that time revealed

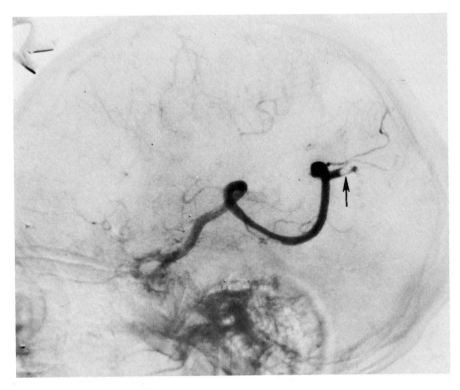

FIG. 1C. A later film shows occlusion of the feeding vessel with stasis of contrast and an intraluminal defect (*arrow*) suggesting thrombosis. The AVM no longer fills.

normal neurologic examination except for a bruit. Arteriogram disclosed a large left frontal lobe AVM supplied by multiple branches of the left middle cerebral artery. The patient's lesion was embolized on four separate occasions over a 6-year period because of severe headaches and increasing neurological deficit. Symptoms were palliated on each occasion following embolization, and subsequent arteriograms showed improved circulation to the normal brain and decreased shunting of blood through the AVM (Fig. 2). A total of 223 spheres (mostly of 1.5 mm diameter) were injected during these procedures without radiographic evidence of any stray pellets. Innumerable radiopaque emboli were noted to be lodged within the interstices of the AVM on plain radiographs. On each occasion the procedure was terminated when the patient experienced neurologic deficits (paresthesia and decreased strength in the right hand). In each instance the deficit was brief, and return to preembolization neurologic status had occurred before the patient left the angiographic table. Long-term follow-up has shown continued disability (headache, seizures, impaired memory), but clinical improvement was documented following each embolization procedure. No permanent deficit occurred as a result of the intervention.

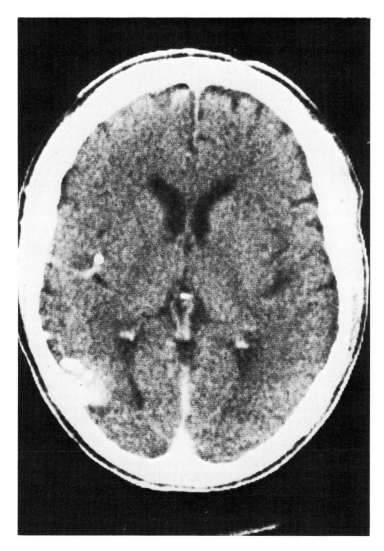

FIG. 1D. A contrast enhanced CT scan done one week after embolization shows opaque emboli within the AVM and one of the errant spheres related to a Sylvian branch vessel.

Case 3: A 30-year-old black male had been asymptomatic until he developed the abrupt onset of left hemiparesis. He was then evaluated and found to have a large right frontoparietal AVM supplied by branches of the ipsilateral anterior and middle cerebral arteries (Fig. 3). For 2 years prior to the present admission he was debilitated with uncontrolled focal motor and grand mal seizures in addition to the left-sided weakness.

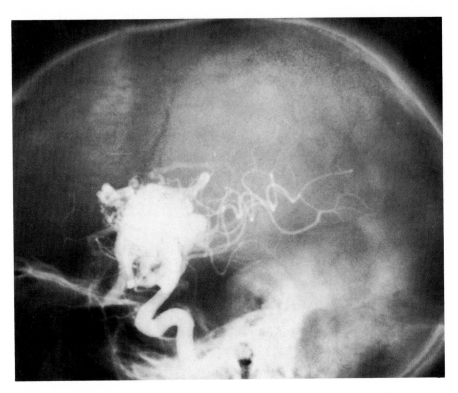

FIG. 2A. Most of the internal carotid supply is shunted into this frontal lobe AVM by multiple dilated middle cerebral artery feeders.

Although the major supply to the AVM was from the anterior cerebral which was considered nonembolizable, attempt was made to embolize the middle cerebral contribution. It was thought that improved perfusion of normal brain might be accomplished by this procedure. Ninety-six pellets 2 mm in diameter were injected into the right internal carotid artery after four initial 1.0-mm spheres went through the AVM into the lungs. The larger spheres occluded multiple branches of the middle cerebral artery including feeders to the AVM as well as several normal branches. The patient had no change in his neurologic status during the procedure. There was indeed a significant reduction in the middle cerebral supply to the AVM, but no change in the size of the AVM was noted. As expected, none of the large anterior cerebral feeders could be embolized, and very few pellets lodged within the AVM itself. The following evening the patient complained of increasing left-sided weakness and numbness. This extension of his deficit had slowly reversed to near preembolization status by the time he was discharged 2 weeks later. Three months later he was readmitted with uncontrollable Jacksonian seizures involving his left arm, leg, and face, and he was noted to be markedly hemiparetic.

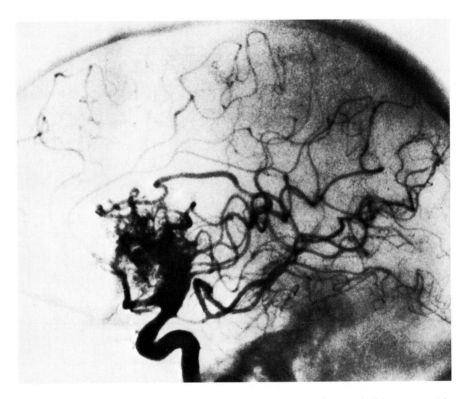

FIG. 2B. An arteriogram following the fourth embolization reveals a marked improvement in anterior, middle, and posterior cerebral perfusion.

Case 4: This 63-year-old man was evaluated for lethargy and pain in his shoulders when a bruit was heard prompting arteriography. This study revealed a left posterior temporal lobe arteriovenous malformation supplied predominantly by the ipsilateral posterior cerebral group. A minor middle cerebral and external carotid supply was also detected (Fig. 4). Selective vertebral angiography was impossible because of tortuosity, origin stenosis, and small arteries bilaterally.

Embolization was attempted with a catheter placed in the left internal carotid. A favorable situation for emboli to enter the AVM from the markedly dilated posterior communicating artery was thought to exist. Thirty-four pellets 1.5 mm in diameter each were injected with initial plain films showing lodging of the opaque spheres within the AVM. The procedure was terminated when the patient suddenly became hemiparetic and aphasic after injection of the 34th embolus. The arteriogram showed diminution in the size of the AVM, and shunting through the lesion was diminished. Improved anterior cerebral territory perfusion was demonstrated. Middle cerebral supply to the AVM was eliminated, but the normal MCA suprasylvian parenchymal branches were also noted to have been affected adversely. The patient's motor

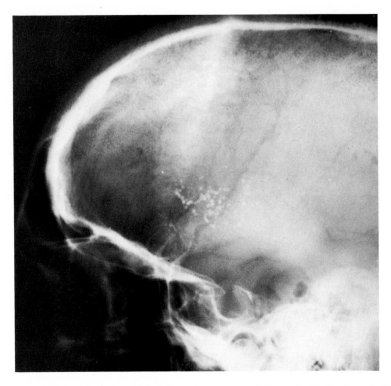

FIG. 2C. A plain radiograph taken early in the process of the patient's fourth embolization shows all opaque spheres to overlie the nidus of the malformation.

strength had returned at time of discharge, but there was still some mild dysphasia.

Case 5: This 10-year-old boy was in excellent health until he experienced a sudden episode of pain in his left shoulder and arm which caused him to fall to the ground. Subsequent examination on his arrival in the emergency room revealed a Brown–Sequard deficit (right-sided pain and temperature loss with a left-sided hemiparesis). The lumbar puncture was bloody. Spinal cord angiography showed the presence of an AVM at the C7 to T1 cord level anterolaterally (Fig. 5).

Embolization was chosen as the treatment best suited for remedy of this lesion (3) and was performed 1 month later at our institution.

Fifteen pellets (0.5 mm each) were employed following selective catherization of the only identified artery of supply (an intercostal branch coming off the left side of the descending aorta at the T5 vertebral level). Puddling and stasis of contrast media was identified fluoroscopically within the AVM during embolization. When the main radicular feeding branch was noted to be occluded on fluoroscopic test injection, arteriogram was obtained and the procedure was terminated. The angio-

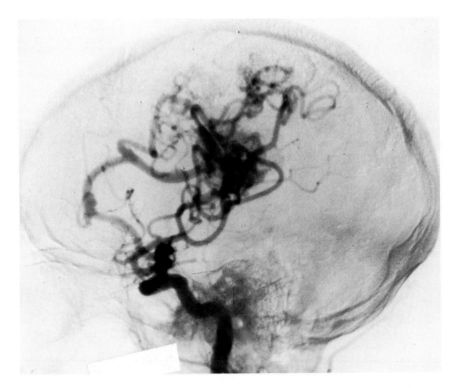

FIG. 3A. A large frontoparietal AVM is supplied by branches from the anterior and middle cerebral arteries.

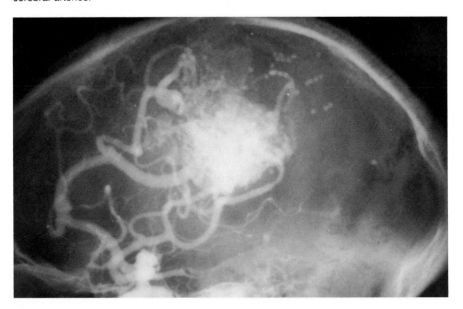

FIG. 3B. The final arteriogram reveals obliteration of much of the middle cerebral supply especially superior to the nidus where pellets are noted lined up in feeding arteries.

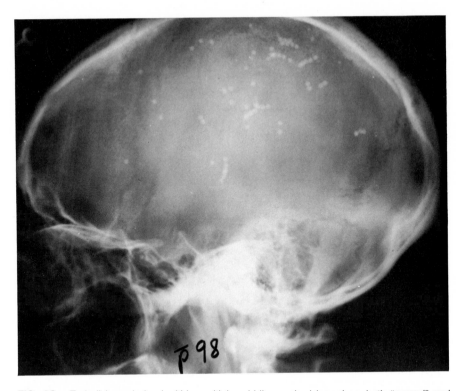

FIG. 3C. Emboli have lodged within multiple middle cerebral branches, both "normal" and abnormal. Very few appear to be within the nidus of the AVM.

gram revealed that the main feeding radicular branch and another much smaller branch feeder had been occluded by emboli. The AVM no longer could be visualized. There was no change in the patient's neurologic status during the procedure. Clinical follow-up 11 months later revealed persistence of the original spastic left hemiparesis with little useful hand function. There was no recurrence of subarachnoid hemorrhage. Repeat angiography at this time showed renewed visualization of the AVM which was 50% of its original size, being supplied by the smaller of the two original feeders that had recanalized and enlarged. The larger original feeder remained nonopacified. It was elected to continue following the patient and to consider reembolization at some undetermined future date.

DISCUSSION

Embolization of cerebral AVMs has been performed at our institution since 1974 in instances where primary surgical resection was not considered to be the treatment of choice. A cure of the AVM can be achieved only by total ablation of the nidus of the AVM. Rarely, if ever, is this possible by means of transcatheter particulate embolization. Palliation of the patient's symptoms, on the other hand, has often been

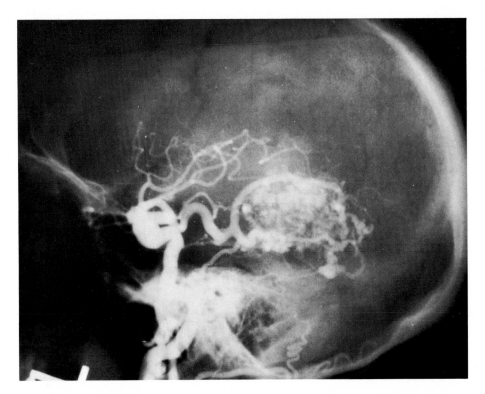

FIG. 4A. This posterior temporal lobe AVM gains its principal supply from the dilated posterior cerebral artery. Blood is shunted away from the middle cerebral territory which shows a marked decrease in perfusion.

achieved, and in numerous cases the size of the AVM has been reduced. Improved circulation to the brain surrounding the AVM results from decreased abnormal shunting after embolization.

When patients have been properly selected, the success of embolization is high and the risk low. The risk of nonintervention, the so-called conservative treatment, must be taken into account also, as this is known to be considerable. The AVM may rupture at any time causing life-threatening subarachnoid hemorrhage. The continued debilitation of the patient related to the presence of the AVM (e.g., uncontrollable seizures, progressive neurological deficits, and severe chronic headaches) may also require the physicians to consider embolization and its risks as a necessary alternative to noninterference in the "natural history" of the condition. In some cases where surgery will be performed, embolization done beforehand to reduce or eliminate portions of the AVM will be effective in making removal simpler and safer than it would otherwise be (7). It might allow the surgeon to approach the lesion from a different, more favorable route if embolization can effectively alter the arterial supply beforehand.

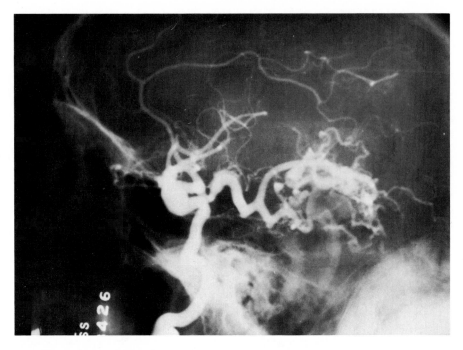

FIG. 4B. Following embolization there is less opacification of the AVM, and the anterior cerebral arteries now fill. Unfortunately the middle cerebral territory now has a further reduction in perfusion caused by stray pellets.

Because this technique does not allow super selective catheterization, the inadvertent embolization of normal branch arteries can and will occur.

The particles, early in the procedures, are almost all drawn into the AVM by the sump effect of the lesion (2,10,11). During embolization, a point is reached when the flow to the normal brain is equal to the flow to the AVM. At this time the risk of stray emboli is significant. The goal is to reduce the size of the AVM as much as possible without the complication of particles going into normal branches. To stop on the conservative side where no emboli have strayed, but where the AVM is only slightly reduced, is being insufficiently aggressive. To stop at the point of maximal obtainable obliteration just before the next embolus enters the normal circulation is the ideal end point. It is improbable that this goal can often be achieved, but it should be closely approximated. Because of the tendency to have stray emboli as the shunt is reduced and the sump effect diminished, one should put up only one particle at a time midway through and later into the procedure. If the first spheres introduced singly have been documented as successfully going into the AVM and the need for many, perhaps hundreds, of particles is anticipated, multiple pellets can safely be injected early in the procedure until the sump effect is altered noticeably. The problem of stray emboli can be minimized with proper selection of patients and attention to details of technique, but a completely safe and yet effective end point remains difficult to achieve.

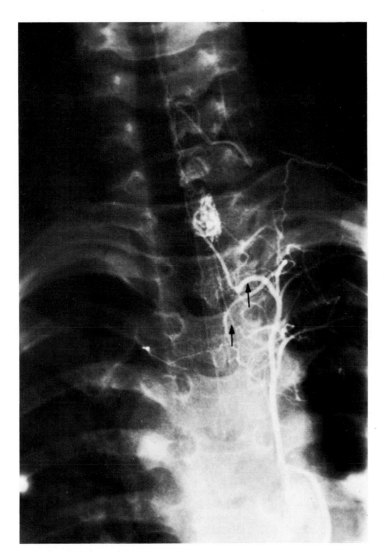

FIG. 5A. An AVM of the spinal cord was found at the cervicothoracic junction supplied by 2 radicular branches *(arrows)* of this intercostal artery.

Silastic pellets are biocompatible and have been used since the early 1960s (4,5,10). The course of travel of the spherical particles is entirely flow-determined after being set free within the circulation. The pellets will generally take the straightest route. They will tend to avoid acute angled branches off the parent artery. If emboli have been put into the internal carotid artery, they will tend to continue into the middle cerebral group rather than entering the anterior cerebral circulation. This is true even if the anterior cerebral is markedly larger in diameter than the middle cerebral (2,6,11). Therefore, AVMs supplied by the middle cerebral artery

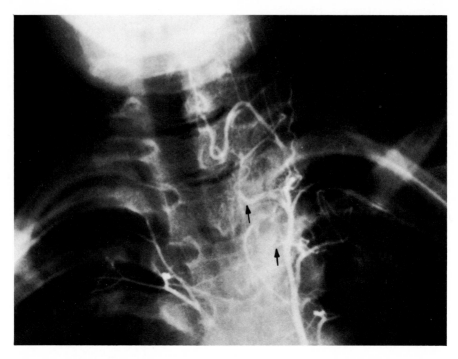

FIG. 5B. Arteriogram immediately following embolization shows no opacification of the AVM. The two vessels of supply have been occluded *(arrows)*.

tend to be easily embolizable from the carotid, whereas those supplied by the anterior cerebral artery are inaccessible and unsafe for this type of embolization. Similarly, the posterior cerebral artery is considered to be the destination of most emboli set free into the vertebral artery. It then follows that those AVMs supplied predominantly by the posterior cerebral artery may be considered embolizable when the catheter is placed selectively within the vertebral artery.

When studying the angiogram prior to embolization, consider that the flow-directed free embolus at any juncture point to the circulation will (a) be drawn toward the AVM by the sump effect of the abnormal shunt, (b) tend to go straight rather than turn, (c) take the branch with the least acute angle off the parent vessel, (d) take the larger vessel (flow depends on the fourth power of the radius), and (e) be affected by a different combination of factors than the preceding embolus. The important sump effect diminishes with each embolus lodging within the AVM or contributing artery. Also, the diameter of feeding vessels may decrease and normal branches increase in size as embolization progresses. AVMs located more distally are less favorable (11), because the embolus has to make more correct choices to get to the lesion than is the case for proximally located lesions. The more tortuous the feeding arteries are (and this may be considerable in these lesions) the more turbulence is created. Therefore, the more random and less predictable becomes the course of emboli traveling therein.

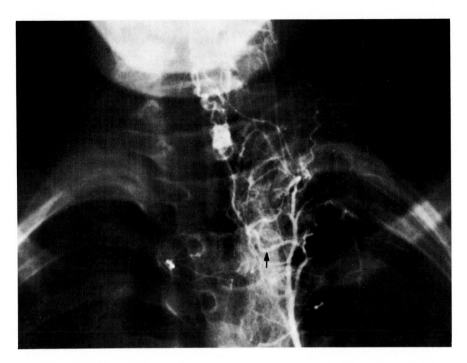

FIG. 5C. Follow-up angiogram approximately 1 year later shows recanalization of a previously occluded radicular branch which again contributes to the AVM. The nidus of the lesion is about 50% of its initial presenting size.

The choice of particle size is critical. Emboli should be large enough to lodge within the AVM without passing through it. Analysis of the arteriogram beforehand may reveal the number and caliber of the draining veins to exceed the number and caliber of the supplying arteries. This situation has been found to be unfavorable for embolization as the fistulous shunts within the AVM nidus are too large for capture of particles (8). A secondary objective becomes embolization of the feeding arteries if embolization of the nidus is impossible. This is analogous to proximal ligation done surgically and is temporary and perhaps futile. Unless all of the feeders can be obliterated, collateral flow to the AVM will always be established at the expense of the normal brain. Following embolization of the nidus itself, however, it may become desirable to continue with larger particles to occlude some of the feeding vessels. The ideal ratio of diameter of feeding arteries to normal branch arteries has been determined to be 4:1 (9,11). Under these conditions particle size may be chosen which will freely enter the feeding branch but which will be too large to stray into the smaller normal branch vessels.

The smooth Silastic spheres are nonthrombogenic. It is this limitation that prevents complete and permanent obliteration of the AVM. Other materials such as Ivalon sponge are thrombogenic and nonabsorbable and may replace Silastic pellets in many cases requiring particulate embolization in the future (1). Gelfoam particles are not employed because they are reabsorbable and produce only temporary occlusion.

Deficits caused by stray pellets are usually temporary. Such errant emboli often lodge in the arteries closely adjacent to the AVM in brain which has been relatively ischemic all along, having been robbed of blood by the AVM. Formation of collateral circuits is potentiated under such circumstances. When the embolization procedure is successful in decreasing the size of the AVM, perfusion in the brain surrounding the AVM is markedly improved. This may more than compensate for blockages from an occasional stray pellet (9,10). Of course, the damage from this complication can be permanent and serious. The frequency of this complication must be minimized, but some risk is certainly justifiable when the alternatives of leaving the lesion to its own devices or operating for surgical removal are judged to present even greater jeopardy.

The procedure may be employed on multiple occasions for palliation of symptoms. It is not known whether embolization reduces the chances of bleeding, but it is generally thought that the potential for bleeding remains as long as any portion of the AVM exists. Pellet embolization may not be trusted to be a curative procedure. Some of the newer modalities, i.e., selective catheterization of feeding arteries with balloon catheters through which bucrylate can be injected to glue the lesion (1), may become curative procedures in some instances. In other cases palliation to a much greater degree than with pellet embolization may be achieved. Such procedures, however, are at present still in the hands of a few highly skilled interventionists using materials not yet available in the United States without special approval. These newer procedures are extremely time consuming as well and may not become practical except in a few centers in this country.

Pellet embolization can be considered a practical and acceptable form of treatment for some AVMs of the brain supplied principally by middle cerebral or posterior cerebral arterial branches. External carotid feeders can also be embolized. Those AVMs whose principal blood supply is from the anterior cerebral group cannot be treated effectively. It is occasionally desirable, however, to embolize the ancillary middle cerebral supply to such malformations.

CONCLUSION

Pellet embolization of central nervous system AVMs may be employed as effective treatment in many instances. Careful assessment of the patient's angiogram together with knowledge of the principles summarized in Table 1 will allow the neuroradiologist to determine whether the patient is a candidate for this type of embolization. One can reasonably expect palliation of symptoms with clinical and angiographic improvement following most embolizations that have been properly selected. The morbidity and mortality is low and within acceptable limits. Although complete eradication of the malformation is not a reasonable expectation, no bridges have been burned for further therapy at some future date. Additional embolization, different types of embolizations, or surgery can still be instituted when needed. The skills of this procedure are basic to more refined embolization techniques. The neuroradiologist can now choose from among a variety of embolic agents and delivery systems to utilize what will work best in a particular instance. As embol-

TABLE 1. *Factors governing the course of a free embolus*

1. Sump effect of the AVM or fistula
2. Tendency to take most direct route
a. Goes straight or takes the branch with the least acute angle from the parent artery
b. Favors least tortuous course
c. MCA is the "end artery" or the continuation of the internal carotid
d. PCA is the "end artery" of the vertebrobasilar system
3. Tendency to follow the branch with the greatest diameter
4. AVM's in the proximal distribution of a major artery more favorable for embolization than those located distally

ization increases in popularity and success for treatment of AVMs, the principles above described will remain invaluable as knowledge fundamental to the interventionist. Pellet embolization will be one of many procedures at his disposal for the most appropriate therapy in any given case. Surgery must still be considered as necessary for any curative effort.

REFERENCES

1. Berenstein, A., and Kricheff, I. (1979): Catheter and material selection for transarterial embolization: Technical considerations. *Radiology*, 132:619–639.
2. Boulos, R., Kricheff, I., and Chase, M. E. (1970): Value of cerebral angiography in the embolization treatment of cerebral arteriovenous malformations. *Radiology*, 97:65–70.
3. Djindjian, R., Cophignon, J., Rey, A., Theron, J., Merland, J. J., and Houdart, R. (1973): Superselective arteriographic embolization by the femoral route in Neuroradiology. Study of 50 cases. II. Embolization in vertebromedullary pathology. *Neuroradiology*, 6:132–143.
4. Kricheff, I., Madayag, M., and Braunstein, P. (1972): Transfemoral catheter embolization of cerebral and posterior fossa arteriovenous malformations. *Radiology*, 103:107–111.
5. Luessenhop, A. J., and Spence, W. T. (1960): Artificial embolization of cerebral arteries: Report of use in a case of arteriovenous malformation. *J.A.M.A.*, 172:1153–1155.
6. Luessenhop, A. J., Kackmann, R., Shevlin, W., and Ferrero, A. A. (1965): Clinical evaluation of artificial embolization in the management of large cerebral arteriovenous malformations. *J. Neurosurg.*, 23:400–417.
7. Luessenhop, A. J., and Presper, J. H. (1975): Surgical embolization of cerebral arteriovenous malformations through internal carotid and vertebral arteries. *J. Neurosurg.*, 42:443–451.
8. Patronas, M. J., Marx, W. J., Duda, E. E., and Mullan, J. J. (1980): Microvascular embolization of arteriovenous malformations: Predicting success by cerebral angiography. *Am. J. Neuroradiol.*, 1:459–462.
9. Stein, B. M., and Wolpert, S. M. (1980): Arteriovenous malformations of the brain. Parts I and II: Current concepts and treatment. *Arch. Neurol.*, 37:1–5, 69–75.
10. Wolpert, S. M., and Stein, B. M. (1975): Catheter embolization of intracranial arteriovenous malformations as an aid to surgical excision. *Neuroradiology*, 10:73–85.
11. Wolpert, S. M., and Stein, B. M. (1979): Factors governing the course of emboli in the therapeutic embolization of cerebral arteriovenous malformations. *Radiology*, 131:125–131.

Vascular Malformations, edited by
R. R. Smith, A. Haerer and W. F. Russell.
Raven Press, New York © 1982.

Intracranial Arteriovenous Malformation with Increased Intracranial Pressure: Response to Embolization

*Thomas A. Tomsick, **John M. Tew, Jr., †Robert R. Lukin, and ††James McLennan

*Departments of *·†Neuroradiology and Neurosurgery, **Good Samaritan and ††University of Cincinnati Hospitals, Cincinnati, Ohio 45220*

Intracranial arteriovenous malformations (AVM) have been reported to cause headache, papilledema, and increased intracranial pressure (5,8,11,12). This is not often seen in the absence of previous hemorrhage or hydrocephalus. Reports have theorized that increased cerebral blood volume or increased dural sinus pressure may cause diminished cerebrospinal fluid (CSF) absorption and increased CSF pressure (3). Combined venous and CSF pressure measurements in AVM have rarely been reported (4,9). We have examined two patients with this syndrome in an attempt to determine the relationship between jugular bulb venous pressure (JBVP) and increased intracranial pressure, and to determine pressure responses to embolization.

Case 1: A 31-year-old white male presented in 1976 complaining of 2 days of right-sided headache and left-sided paresthesia. He had an 8-year history of episodic numbness, tingling, and questionable weakness which had spread from his fingertips to his shoulder. The episodes lasted approximately 30 min. Approximately 3 years prior to admission, right frontal and temporal throbbing headaches associated with nausea and vomiting and photophobia followed the episodes of numbness and tingling.

Physical examination revealed blurred disc margins bilaterally, absent venous pulsations, but no hemorrhages or exudates. There was no meningismus. A lumbar puncture was not performed initially. Angiography demonstrated a large AVM in the parietal region of the right hemisphere, fed primarily by the right middle cerebral artery (Fig. 1).

Over the next 3 years, the patient's visual acuity diminished to 20/400 in the right eye. Constriction of the visual fields was also documented. Lumbar puncture revealed an opening pressure of 220 cm of water.

By July of 1979, the patient's visual acuity had diminished to 20/100 O.S., and finger counting at 1 meter O.D. Bilateral papilledema was again present. Lumbar pressure was 440 mm of water. Jugular bulb pressure was measured at 14 mm Hg. Embolization of the AVM with 200 Silastic beads (1.5 and 2.0 mm) resulted in incomplete obliteration of the vascular malformation (Fig. 1, C and D). Jugular bulb venous pressure decreased to 5 mm Hg within 24 hr. The patient felt improved

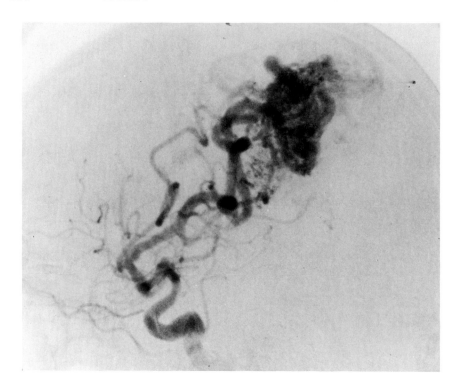

FIG. 1A. Preembolization right common carotid angiogram, lateral view. Enlarged posterior frontal and parietal branches of the middle cerebral artery fill the AVM.

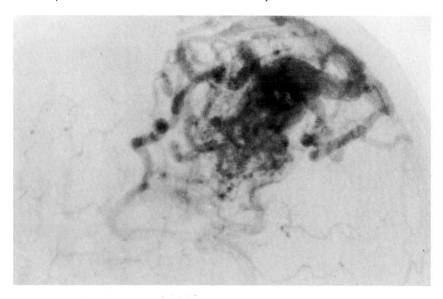

FIG. 1B. Preembolization. Venous phase, 1 sec later.

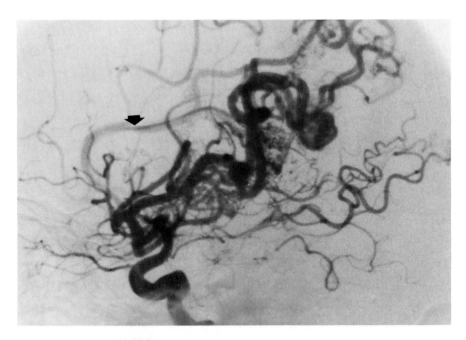

FIG. 1C. Postembolization right internal carotid angiogram. An arterial phase film at approximately the same stage of filling of **Fig. 1A**. The anterior cerebral fills faintly *(arrow)*. There is delayed opacification of the sinusoids of the AVM, despite greater filling of the distal cortical branches.

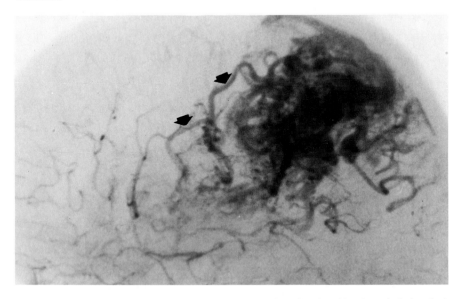

FIG. 1D. Postembolization. Venous phase, 1 sec later. Slow flow is evident in occluded cortical branches *(arrows)*. The largest draining vein still opacifies the sagittal sinus, but there is delayed appearance of other cortical veins.

after embolization with some decrease in headaches and subjective improvement of vision.

Case 2: A 38-year-old male complained of headaches of 2 years' duration, with increasing severity. He also complained of a noise behind his right ear, which was causing difficulty in concentration. Angiography performed at another hospital showed a dural AVM chiefly supplied by the right occipital artery, right posterior auricular artery, with less supply from the right middle meningeal artery and meningohypophysial trunk (Fig. 2A). Some cross filling and contribution from the opposite external carotid artery was also present.

Physical examination on admission showed blurred disc margins bilaterally. Venous pulsations were present. A right retromastoid bruit and thrill were present.

Lumbar puncture pressure was not performed, but an isotope cisternogram demonstrated rapid appearance of radiopharmaceutical in the basal cisterns at 4 hr, with delayed flow over the convexity at 24 and 48 hr (Fig. 2B). A CT scan showed borderline-size lateral ventricles. The JBVP was 21 mm Hg systolic, with a mean of 18 mm Hg.

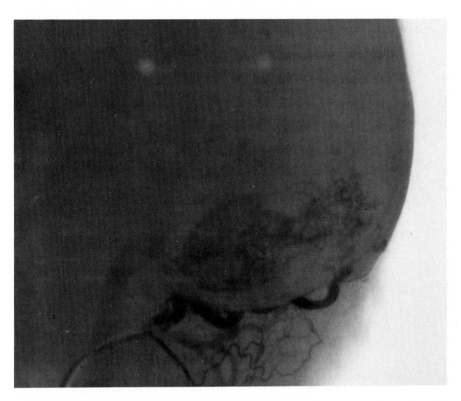

FIG. 2A. Selective right occipital artery injection reveals multiple penetrating branches with shunting to the transverse and sigmoid sinuses.

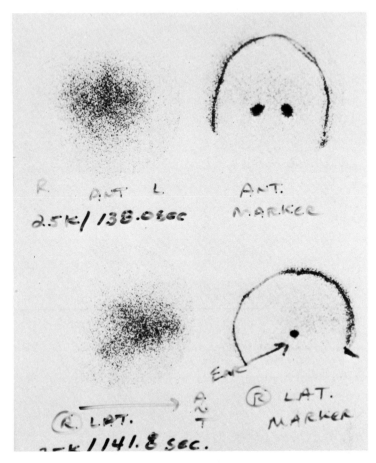

FIG. 2B. 24-hr [169]Yb cisternogram shows radiopharmaceutical in the basilar cisterns, sylvian cistern, and interhemispheric region, but delayed concentration over the parasagittal convexity.

Embolization of the right occipital artery with polyvinyl alcohol foam was performed on 2/29/80 (Fig. 2C).

On 4/15/80, the patient was readmitted for further embolization. Headaches had diminished in the interim, but a bruit was still heard over the right retromastoid region. Occlusion of the left occipital artery, and occlusion of the right posterior auricular artery was performed. Incomplete occlusion of numerous superficial temporal artery branches on the right and further occlusion of the right occipital artery was performed. The patient heard no bruit, and had no headaches within 24 hr of the procedure. The audible bruit had disappeared.

The patient was readmitted 6/12/80. The patient had had no interval headaches, and heard no bruits. Repeat angiography demonstrated some persistent flow to the

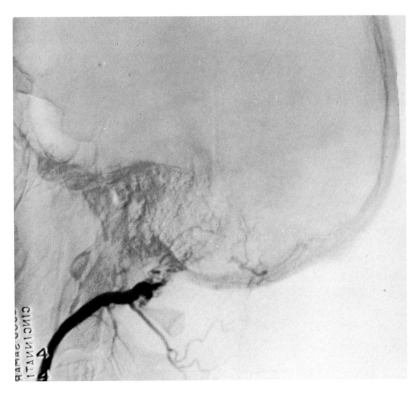

FIG. 2C. Occluded right occipital artery following polyvinyl alcohol embolization (2/29/80).

malformation via now hypertrophied branches of the external carotid artery (Fig. 2D). Further embolization of these vessels was performed. A postembolization study of the right common carotid demonstrated marked reduction in flow to the transverse sinus malformation, primarily by distal branches of the right middle meningeal artery, and distal collateral branches from the right superficial temporal artery (Fig. 2E). Two months following the last embolization, the patient complained of no headaches or noise, and no bruit was heard. There was no evidence of papilledema.

DISCUSSION

A reduced CSF absorption syndrome has been defined by considering factors controlling CSF absorption: The pressure gradient between the subarachnoid space and the superior sagittal sinus ($P_{CSF} - P_{SS}$) might be expected with AVMs having large shunts at high pressure to the venous circulation. Physiologic studies in cases of AVM with increased intracranial pressure are lacking. Normal sagittal sinus and torcular pressures are given by Milhorat as 9.0 and 4.6 cm saline, respectively, based on the work of Shulman (6,10).

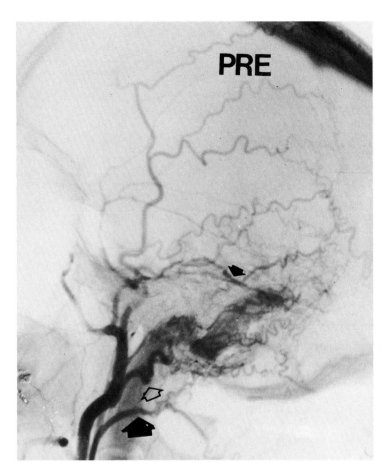

FIG. 2D. Right external carotid artery angiogram (6/12/80). Partially recanalized occipital artery *(large closed arrow)*, posterior auricular artery *(open arrow)*, middle meningeal artery *(small closed arrow)*, and superficial temporal artery branches are shunting to the transverse and sigmoid sinus.

The JBVP in Case 2 at 21.0 mm Hg was clearly elevated. The clinical findings indicating increased intracranial pressure were compelling. Cerebrospinal fluid pressure was not measured at the time of isotope injection for cisternography. The isotope cisternogram showing delayed passage of radiopharmaceutical over the convexity suggests a delayed pattern of CSF flow and absorption. Although the pressure measurements and cisternogram were not repeated postembolization, the clinical improvement leads us to conclude the syndrome was reversed by embolization.

Case 1 exhibited a less elevated JBVP which did decrease postembolization. This pressure reduction was obtained despite only subtle angiographic evidence of flow reduction postembolization.

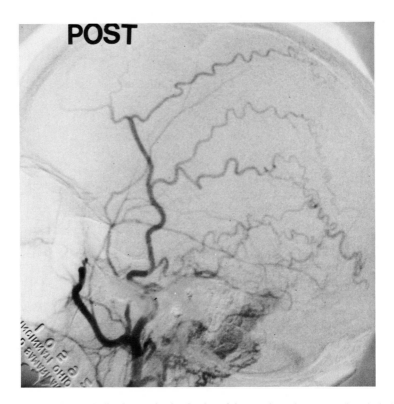

FIG. 2E. Following embolization, reduction in size of the meningeal artery, and occluded flow in the occipital and posterior auricular arteries lead to marked reduction in opacification of the sinus.

Our experience does not prove that increased blood volume or increased sinus pressure directly caused increased CSF pressure. In the case of the dural AVM, it is suggested that increased dural sinus pressure was the etiologic mechanism. Papilledema has been recognized in 15 out of 86 cases of transverse sinus AVMs, a number of which were associated with some degree of occlusion or thrombosis of the sinus (1,3). Increased blood volume could be operative in the case of a cerebral AVM in combination with direct sinus pressure alterations.

Recent intraoperative measurements of AVM draining vein pressure have been performed by Nornes. None of the patients in his series were reported to have increased intracranial pressure. Cortical venous pressures ranged from 8 to 23 mm Hg, and sinus pressures were not reported (7).

This interesting problem offers fertile ground for further clinical investigation of CSF dynamics with AVMs. The role of surgical extirpation, embolization, CSF drainage procedures, or medical management is yet to be elucidated. It is suggested, however, that some degree of control of elevated pressure may be offered by such vascular occlusive techniques.

REFERENCES

1. Houser, O. W., Campbell, J. K., Campbell, R. J., and Sundt, T. M. (1979): Arteriovenous malformation affecting the transverse dural venous sinus—An acquired lesion. *Mayo Clin. Proc.*, 54:651–661.
2. Johnston, I. (1973): Reduced CSF absorption syndrome. *Lancet*, 2:418–420.
3. Kuhner, A., Krastel, A., and Stoll, W. (1976): Arteriovenous malformations of the transverse sinus. *J. Neurosurg.*, 45:12–19.
4. Lamase, Lobato, R. D., Esparza, J., and Esludero, L. (1977): Dural posterior fossa AVM producing raised sagittal sinus pressure. *J. Neurosurg.*, 46:810.
5. Michelson, W. J. (1978): Natural history and pathophysiology of arteriovenous malformation. *Clin. Neurosurg.*, 27:307–313.
6. Milhorat, T. H. (1972): *Hydrocephalus and the Cerebrospinal Fluid.* Williams and Wilkins Company, Baltimore, Maryland.
7. Nornes, H., and Grip, A. (1980): Hemodynamic aspects of cerebral arteriovenous malformations. *J. Neurosurg.*, 53:456–464.
8. Paterson, J. H., and McKissock, W. (1956): A clinical survey of intracranial angiomas with special reference to their mode of progression and surgical treatment: A report of 110 cases. *Brain*, 79:233–266.
9. Shenkin, H. A., Spitz, E. B., Grant, F. C., and Kety, S. S. (1948): Physiologic studies of arteriovenous anomalies of the brain. *J. Neurosurg.*, 5:165–172.
10. Shulman, K., Yarnell, P., and Ransohoff, J. (1964): Dural sinus pressure in normal and hydrocephalic dogs. *Arch. Neurol.*, 10:560–575.
11. Vassilouthis, J. (1979): Cerebral arteriovenous malformation with intracranial hypertension. *Surg. Neurol.*, 11:402–404.
12. Weisberg, C. A., Peirce, J. F., and Jabbari, B. (1977): Intracranial hypertension resulting from a cerebrovascular malformation. *South. Med. J.*, 10:624–626.
13. Young, B. (1979): Hydrocephalus and elevated intracranial pressure. *Child's Brain*, 5:73–80.

Vascular Malformations, edited by
R.R. Smith, A. Haerer and W.F. Russell.
Raven Press, New York © 1982.

Combined Neurosurgical-Neuroradiological Therapy for Cerebral Arteriovenous Malformations—The Walter Reed Protocol

Eugene D. George and Paul H. Pevsner

Departments of Neurosurgery and Neuroradiology, Walter Reed Army Medical Center, Washington, D.C. 20012

Large numbers of patients with cerebral arteriovenous malformations (AVM) are currently being evaluated at Walter Reed Army Medical Center. Many of these patients have lesions previously thought either unresectable or resectable only with unacceptably high risks for devastating morbidity. The development of intravascular embolization techniques now allows conversion of these AVMs to surgically resectable lesions. The technique utilized at Walter Reed involves intravascular delivery via a mini-balloon catheter of isobutyl-2-cyanoacrylate[1] to the interstices of the AVM (5,6,8,9,12–14).

Acrylic embolization can be accomplished either by percutaneous angiographic techniques with super selective mini-balloon catheterization or direct intraoperative injection of exposed feeding vessels.

A protocol was developed for the treatment and serial follow-up evaluations of such patients. Patient evaluation is a combined team approach by the principal investigators from the Neurosurgery and Neuroradiology Services. Such cooperation is essential to provide optimal care to these high-risk patients. All selected patients presented with either intracranial hemorrhage, seizures, progressive neurologic deficit, or these in some combination. At present, headaches alone are not considered sufficient indication for therapy.

The therapeutic goal is total ablation of the AVM, not merely occlusion of feeding vessels or decrease in angioma size. If the lesion is not completely obliterated and/or resected, a valid question exists whether any significant treatment has occurred. The goal of AVM polymerization is total obliteration of interstices, not merely decrease in AVM size. However, less than total obliteration of AVM interstices may be sufficient in patients when polymerization techniques are used solely as adjuncts to facilitate surgical resection.

All patients seen at Walter Reed with intracranial AVMs meeting the criteria are offered a specific recommended therapeutic approach involving either direct mi-

---

The statements contained in this paper are the opinions of the authors, and do not in any way or manner reflect on the Walter Reed Army Medical Center or the Department of the Army.

---

[1]Ethicon, Inc., Somerville, New Jersey.

129

crosurgical resection or combined intravascular polymerization with probable subsequent surgical resection. Protocol exceptions include certain low-flow, small deep lesions, elderly patients presenting with seizures alone, or patients with other medical conditions precluding aggressive therapy.

It must be stressed that AVM polymerization techniques are reserved solely for patients with extremely high-risk lesions. The large number of such patients (11 of 24 during the first 10 months of study) being seen at Walter Reed reflects the specific referral of highly screened patients from other Army neurosurgical centers. All AVMs appearing surgically resectable by optimal microsurgical techniques are so resected without adjunctive use of polymerization techniques.

The Walter Reed Protocol presently dictates surgical resection following AVM polymerization. This is carried out several months postpolymerization to allow resolution of brain swelling and delayed spontaneous AVM obliteration occasionally seen (5 of 11 patients embolized). Arteriovenous malformations lying in deep critical areas of the brain which have been obliterated by embolization techniques alone are not routinely resected. These patients will be followed with serial angiography at prearranged intervals over future years.

This report describes the results and complications in 24 patients treated at Walter Reed Army Medical Center over the previous 10 months through January, 1981. Three additional patients were seen with large AVMs presenting either asymptomatically or with moderate headaches as their sole complaint, determined by computerized tomography (CT) scan and/or angiography. These patients were not included in this study and have not been further treated at Walter Reed. (They will be followed with the treated patients in an attempt to learn more regarding AVM natural history.)

MATERIALS AND METHODS

The techniques, catheter materials, and delivery system used for super-selective intracerebral vascular catheterization and embolization have been described previously (12,14). All patients are evaluated with high-speed cerebral angiography (4–6 films/sec) utilizing simultaneous biplane filming techniques and Conray 60 as the contrast medium. Number 5 French polyethylene catheters are used for selected catheterization of the internal carotid and vertebral arteries with appropriate subtraction views reproduced for adequate evaluation and study.

The patients selected for combined preoperative and/or intraoperative embolization followed by surgical resection are admitted to Walter Reed Army Medical Center several days in advance of the embolization procedure. During this period detailed counseling with patients and their families is carried out by the principal investigators. At this time the patients and their families are informed of the natural history of the disease, and alternative forms of therapy, complications, the experience at Walter Reed Army Medical Center, and their expectation regarding long-term follow-up and therapeutic results.

The percutaneous mini-balloon catheter embolization procedures are carried out in the Angiography Suite. Following scout films and a percutaneous femoral puncture, a preliminary angiogram is performed immediately prior to each embolization procedure. This provides additional information regarding spontaneous resolution or further expansion of the AVM. The mini-balloon catheter is then positioned in the distal appropriate feeding vessel. Anteroposterior and lateral control films are obtained for position localization. The acrylic is then injected (isobutyl-2-cyanoacrylate) and the mini-balloon catheter rapidly removed. An immediate rapid-sequence postembolization angiogram is performed.

Initially, 0.5 cc of acrylic was used for the injections, suspended between two aliquots of sterile water. After careful evaluation of many embolizations, it became clear that smaller volumes delivered multiple times through the feeding vessels were far more effective. In this way interstices were filled and occluded, and there was no abrupt occlusion of the feeding vessel. The abrupt sudden occlusion of a feeding vessel is absolutely contraindicated in the treatment of these lesions unless it occurs retrogradely secondary to complete obliteration of the AVM interstices. The feeding vessel must be kept open as long as possible, allowing it to function as a conduit for further delivery of acrylic. This principle is extremely important in effective ablation of these lesions.

In any session one to three injections of acrylic will be performed. The end point is empiric. If there are any signs of ischemia the procedure is aborted. Several sessions are usually required. The patients are sent home after an observation period of 3 to 10 days and return at weekly to monthly intervals. Some patients have been embolized at weekly intervals and remain hospitalized until completion of embolization.

In a previous report (13), a therapeutic trial of temporary balloon inflation sufficient to cause temporary occlusion of the feeding vessel was advocated to evaluate neurologic deficit to be anticipated if total vascular occlusion of the vessel should occur. Although this maneuver may be of value in some cases, the absence of neurologic symptoms during such balloon inflation in no way guarantees patient tolerance for the embolization procedure.

The operative procedure, carried out under general anesthesia, consists of an appropriately located craniotomy over the feeding vessel or vessels. This vessel complex is exposed microsurgically and cannulated with a small polyethylene catheter passed distally into the lesion. This precludes the undesirable proximal feeding vessel occlusion before delivery of adequate amounts of acrylic into the AVM interstices.

When the feeding vessel can be exposed as it enters the malformation, it can be readily cannulated with a bent 25-gauge needle attached to a tuberculin syringe, and the acrylic injected directly. This method has the sole advantage of being much faster and simpler, converting a maneuver of potentially 30 min into one of 30 sec.

If multiple feeding vessels are to be glued intraoperatively, a large craniotomy flap is reflected, to allow for possible immediate AVM resection should an unexpected major hemorrhage occur. This then becomes the craniotomy flap for possible subsequent surgical resection of the malformation. Thus far, hemorrhage has not occurred, probably as a consequence of the decision to limit intraoperative glueing to partially obliterated AVMs with limited remaining feeder vessels.

Immediately after intraoperative acrylic embolization, high-speed biplane angiography is performed with the patient still under general anesthesia. This involves transferring these patients to the Angiography Suite adjacent to the operating room on completion of wound closure. Because of equipment limitations and accessibility of optimal angiography adjacent to the operating room, intraoperative angiography was not carried out in these patients prior to vessel embolization or as an intraoperative adjunct to surgical resection in the patient having direct surgical resection. It is anticipated that, with the arrival of appropriate equipment, intraoperative angiography will become routine.

Finally, a brief note should be added regarding the methods utilized in patients having a direct microsurgical resection without adjunctive polymerization. These patients were operated with the conventional large craniotomy flaps. Exposure and resections were carried out with optimal microsurgical techniques already well described (7,10,11). Classical methods of malformation resection were utilized, involving careful detailed exposure and control of feeding vessels with preservation of draining veins until late in the procedure. Occasionally, additional use of hypotension, either generalized with the aid of appropriate anesthetic techniques, or localized with temporary occlusion of main vessel trunks from which feeding vessels exited, was utilized. Microsurgical resections of malformations were carried out in slow painstaking fashion with progressive mobilization and malformation diminution in size as the resection progressed. At the conclusion of the resection, the area was thoroughly visualized to ensure persistence of appropriate main cerebral feeding trunks together with resection of any residual malformation. Immediately following closure, with the patient still under general anesthesia, detailed angiography was carried out; this allowed return of the patient to the operating room if evidence of small residual malformation were noted. Frequently, when the resection process had been quite lengthy, immediate angiography was omitted. In these cases early angiography was carried out several days later. If residual AVM was demonstrated, a second surgical resection was performed (Case 2). In all cases where no evidence of residual malformation was visualized, repeat angiography was carried out 4 to 6 months later.

RESULTS

Under this protocol, a total of 24 patients with intracranial intravenous malformations was treated.

Table 1 summarizes the group of 11 patients treated with preoperative and/or intraoperative acrylic embolization with or without postembolization resection of their lesion. It must be stressed that this is a group of extremely high-risk patients, all of whom were considered to be otherwise inoperable by several neurosurgeons in accordance with the protocol. The age range of the combined therapy group was 15 to 55 years with a mean of 29 years. Five patients in the treated group had no immediate or long-term complications directly or indirectly as a result of the embolization. The remaining 6 patients had various neurologic sequelae, including coma, homonymous hemianopsia, dysphasia, and hemiplegia. Most of these episodes were transient, but several of the patients had more than one episode of neurological sequelae following separate embolization procedures. In one patient the distal portions of two mini-balloon catheters were glued into the lesion during sequential embolizations; since the patient suffered no neurological sequelae the catheters were left in place pending a decision regarding removal at the definitive surgical resection. Two patients had associated aneurysms, one bilateral. Three aneurysms were clipped prior to definitive AVM embolization. A patient with a large anterior communicating aneurysm suffered a mild organic brain syndrome in the postoperative period following his aneurysm clipping which, although slowly resolving, resulted in deferring further treatment of his huge dominant hemisphere malformation until further recovery. The other patient tolerated surgical clipping of his bilateral internal carotid aneurysm, but developed dysphasia and marked hemiparesis during the second stage percutaneous mini-balloon polymerization of his large dominant fronto-parietal AVM. Two patients with large dominant hemisphere deep occipital temporal AVMs developed seemingly permanent homonymous hemianopsias. There were no deaths in this group of extremely high-risk patients.

In only 1 case was the permanent deficit sufficiently bothersome to cause either the patient or his physicians to regret treating the patient. Even this patient with significant hemiparesis and mild dysphasia continues to improve steadily.

Table 2 summarizes the group of 13 patients treated solely by microsurgical resection. The age range of patients in this group was 15 to 46 years with a mean of 30 years. This series basically consisted of those patients usually treated by neurosurgeons in centers treating significant numbers of AVMs. Most of those patients had malformations of specific locations, size, or accessibility of feeding vessels as to appear surgically resectable. Other patients had large poorly located AVMs but presented following hemorrhage with sufficient size hematomas to warrant evacuation and AVM resection at that time. A few of these malformations were of significant size and location, including large malformations in the dominant Sylvian fissure, or deep temporal occipital region, as to warrant polymerization therapy. However, these cases demonstrated certain specific characteristics, such as main branches of important feeding vessels coursing through massive angiomas. Another patient, presenting with hemorrhage, had previous Silastic sphere embolization significantly limiting the conduit vessels available for mini-balloon or surgical acrylic polymerization techniques.

One death occurred in this series, a young man with a deep nondominant huge temporal occipital malformation with multiple feeders from the right posterior cerebral and middle cerebral artery branches. This patient presented early in the protocol series during a time when difficulties existed in obtaining isobutyl-2-cyanoacrylate. It was elected to proceed with direct microsurgical resection. During the surgical resection clipping of the feeding vessels and mobilization of the malformation were carried out in a relatively rapid and uneventful fashion. Massive bleeding suddenly occurred during mobilization of a group of draining veins, close to the anticipated termination of the procedure. Despite extensive efforts, diffuse bleeding continued with brain swelling and the patient died. At postmortem examination, a major

TABLE 1. Combined therapy

			Embolizations		Neurological sequelae	
Age/Sex	Location	Presentation	Percutaneous	Direct-surgical	Transient	Permanent
55M	Dominant Left frontal with associated huge comm. artery aneurysm	Seizures	1	1	None	Mild organic brain syndrome—improving (Postop. aneurysm clipping)
31M	Dominant Left parietotemporal	Seizures	2	1	Coma 12 hr postembolization, right hemiparesis with postintraoperative embolization, dyslexia	Mild right hemiparesis, mild dyslexia—improving' homonymous hemianopsia
33F	Dominant Left occipitotemporal	Hemorrhage and seizures	3		Hemiparesis, dysphasia, homonymous hemianopsia	Hemiparesis—improving; homonymous hemianopsia, mild dyslexia—improving
17M	Dominant Left occipitotemporal	Hemorrhage	1		Homonymous hemianopsia	Homonymous hemianopsia
19F	Right parietofrontal	Recurrent hemorrhage, episodic hemiparesis secondary to cerebral steal	3	1	Hemiparesis PG No. 2, mild organic brain syndrome	Minimal hemiparesis

32M	Right frontal with multiple large deep and superficial feeders	Seizures	1	None	None
15F	Midline thalamic	Hemorrhage with seizures	1	Mild left hemi-palgesia below T10	None
22M	Dominant Left frontoparietal	Seizures	1	None	None
38M	Dominant Left frontoparietal	Seizures, hemorrhage, subdural	4	None	None
19M	Nondominant right parietotemporal	Seizures	4	None	None
34M	Dominant Left frontoparietal with associated bilateral comm. artery aneurysms	Hemorrhage	2	Hemiplegia and aphasia	Hemiparesis with dysphasia—improving

TABLE 2. *AVM patients treated surgically only*

| Age/Sex | Location | Presentation | Neurological sequelae | | Mortality |
			Transient	Permanent	
28F	Dominant Frontoparietal intraventricular with hydrocephalus and hematoma	Hemorrhage	Right hemiparesis	Mild right hemiparesis[a]	0
34F	Nondominant Parietooccipital with hematoma and unrelated hematoma	Hemorrhage	Moderate left hemiparesis	Left homonymous hemianopsia[a]	0
21M	Dominant Frontal lobe	Hemorrhage with seizures	None		0
23M	Nondominant Frontoparietal with hematoma	Hemorrhage	Left hemiparesis with parietal sensory deficit and left homonymous hemianopsia	Left homonymous hemianopsia with mild left hemiparesis[a]	0
43F	Nondominant Temporal	Seizures	Moderate organic brain syndrome with labile affect and homonymous hemianopsia	Left homonymous hemianopsia[a]	0

38F	Dominant Frontotemporal	Hemorrhage with seizures	Right hemiparesis with dysphasia, moderate	Mild right hemiparesis with minimal dysphasia[a]	0
35F	Dominant Frontotemporal basal ganglia	Seizures, hemorrhage, recurring hemiparesis with organic mental syndrome	Right hemiparesis with dysphasia, mild	Same[a]	0
23M	Nondominant temporal	Seizures	Homonymous hemianopsia	Homonymous hemianopsia	0
15M	Dominant Parietal temporal	Seizures	None	None	0
32M	Interhemispheric Nondominant Fronto-parietal	Hemorrhage	Moderate left leg spasticity	None[a]	0
31F	Non dominant temporal frontal	Increased ICP with papilledema	Left homonymous quadrantanopsia	Same	0
23M	Nondominant Parietal temporal Occipital	Seizures with probable hemorrhage	Intraoperative death		1
46M	Dominant Frontoparietal	Seizures	Right hemiparesis with dysphasia	None	0

[a]Reflect preoperative status.

feeding arterial complex was found intact, arising deeply from the right posterior cerebral artery proximally in a location obscured by a clump of large draining veins.

Of the remaining patients, the majority had significant transient neurologic deficits, usually reflecting their preoperative status. The permanent sequelae cannot yet be fully evaluated, but they appear limited to homonymous hemianopsia or quadrantanopsia in all but 3 patients; these patients are anticipated to continue their steady improvement over the next year. Detailed long-term follow-up psychometric studies will be carried out.

All of these patients have had total malformation resection determined by follow-up angiography.

DISCUSSION

Large malformations with multiple large feeding vessels coming off the proximal posterior cerebral branches are now routinely embolized with acrylic via mini-balloon catheters prior to surgical resection, converting their resection into a rather simple and uneventful procedure. The death of 1 patient early in the protocol series provided motivation toward rigorous application of the combined approach in succeeding patients. In addition, optimal intraoperative angiography following presumed clipping of the major feeders would have been extremely helpful at the stage just prior to final mobilization in patients with such large and diffuse malformations.

Five patients in the combined intravascular occlusive group subsequently underwent delayed spontaneous thrombosis of all or part of the angioma days to weeks after the mini-balloon embolization. Four of these patients reported headache and slight neck stiffness approximately 2 weeks after embolization. These were all discrete, identifiable events which were entirely separate from the embolizations. A CT scan showed no evidence of repeat hemorrhage in these patients. The mechanism appears to be conversion of high-flow to low-flow lesions. Apparently, there is a critical level of flow below which such occlusions will occur in certain patients.

Intracerebral hemorrhage did not occur in any of these patients during embolization. This is always an area of concern, and is due to either rupture of the feeding vessel by the mini-balloon, or venous outflow occlusion. Arterial feeder vessel rupture has been reported with the Kerber calibrated leak balloon, and is due to local overdistention of the vessel (1,4, A. Berenstein and R. Ethier, *personal communication*). Three years prior to this study a patient undergoing mini-balloon embolization had a sudden intracerebral hemorrhage and died. At post-mortem examination no discrete vessel rupture was identified, nor could it be explained by the conduct of the procedure (13). However, modifications in the mini-balloon were made such that rupture of the balloon would occur at less than 2 lb/in^2 inflation pressure precluding any vessel rupture (14). Isobutyl-2-cyanoacrylate polymerization retardant with iophendylate (Pantopaque®)[2] (4) can result in polymerization of the polymer in the draining veins rather than interstices of the AVM (1, A.

---

[2]Lafayette Pharmacol, Inc., Lafayette, Indiana.

Berenstein and R. Ethier, *personal communication*). A further disadvantage of Pantopaque® and Tantalum is the artifacts introduced in CT scans. This is a critical objection because CT is an absolute adjunct in the follow-up clinical care and evaluation of these patients. For these reasons no radiopaque additives or polymerization retardants are used.

One additional observation became apparent following review of the angiograms with increasing numbers of patients. Those patients who developed hemiparesis or other major neurologic sequelae following embolization, usually after several previous stages of embolization, had already had conversion of high-flow to a low-flow lesion in their malformation. When the malformation was essentially fed from that major vessel region, whether middle cerebral or pericallosal, the last injection resulted in retrograde thrombosis of major feeding vessels at the time of embolization. Following recognition of this phenomenon, lesser amounts of acrylic (0.2 rather than 0.5 cc) were used during this stage of the embolization.

It should be noted that the mini-balloon catheter and delivery system used was developed by the senior neuroradiologist. Furthermore, the catheter approach to acrylic embolization of these patients was based on his personal experience in over 128 head and neck lesions and 72 peripheral lesions treated previously (13,14).

CASE REPORTS

Case 1 (Fig. 1, A–W): A 31-year-old male presented with seizures secondary to a deep parietotemporal dominant hemisphere angioma filling from branches of the left anterior cerebral, middle cerebral, and posterior cerebral arteries. After percutaneous embolization through feeding branches from the left posterior cerebral artery, a significant decrease in size of the angioma was noted. No immediate neurologic sequelae occurred. Approximately 12 hr postembolization his level of consciousness abruptly deteriorated and he developed respiratory distress. An emergency CT scan demonstrated acute ventricular dilation secondary to a mass effect and compression of the posterior third ventricle and aqueduct. A ventricular drain

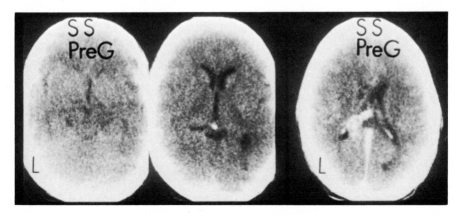

FIG. 1A. Preembolization CT scan (PreG). Pre- and postcontrast scan. Parietotemporal AVM.

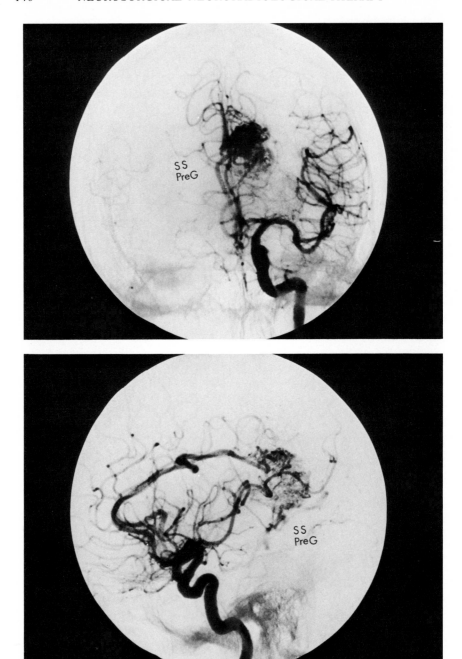

FIG. 1B (top) and **C** (bottom).   Preembolization (PreG). Left internal carotid angiogram (AP and lateral). The AVM is fed by the distal pericallosal artery.

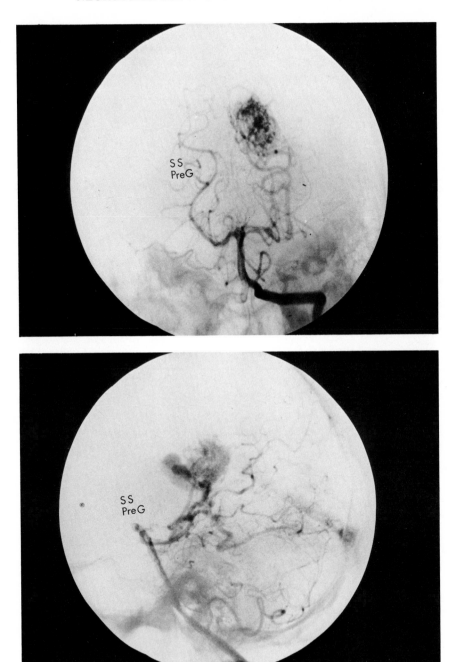

FIG. 1D (top) and **E** (bottom). Preembolization (PreG). Left vertebral angiogram (AP and lateral). The AVM is fed by the left posterior cerebral artery.

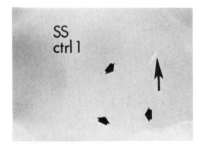
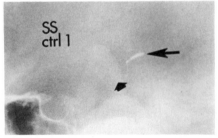

FIG. 1F.   Control miniature balloon position views (Ctrl 1) AP and lateral. The miniature balloon catheter is positioned in the left distal posterior cerebral artery *(arrow)*.

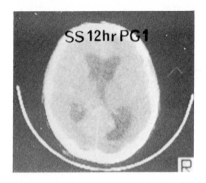

FIG. 1G.   CT scan 12 hr post first embolization (12 hr PG 1).

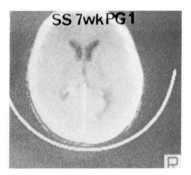

FIG. 1H.   CT scan 7 weeks post first embolization (7 Wk PG 1).

resulted in gradual recovery of consciousness. A transient right hemiparesis and dysphasia cleared over subsequent days. There was no evidence of hemorrhage on CT scan and the mass gradually decreased, allowing removal of the ventriculostomy. A CT scan 7 weeks later showed normal ventricles. A second stage embolization of the distal pericallosal feeding vessels was unsuccessful; the mini-balloon could not be passed beyond A2. Later the distal pericallosal artery was cannulated intra-operatively and the catheter threaded to the malformation region where isobutyl-2-cyanoacrylate, 0.5 cc, was injected. The immediate postsurgical angiogram showed almost no residual angioma. Angiography 2 months later demonstrated significant

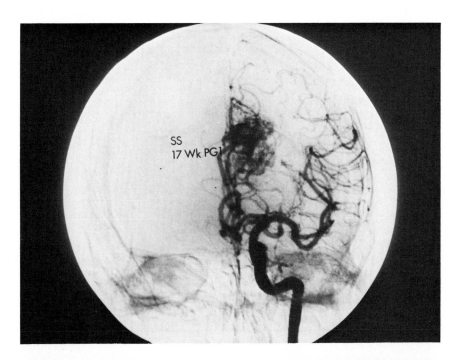

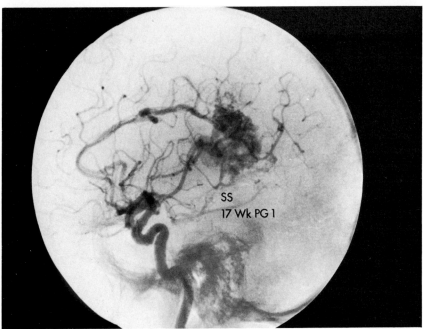

FIG. 1I (top) and **J** (bottom).   Seventeen weeks post first embolization (17 Wk PG 1) left internal carotid angiogram (AP and lateral). Residual AVM.

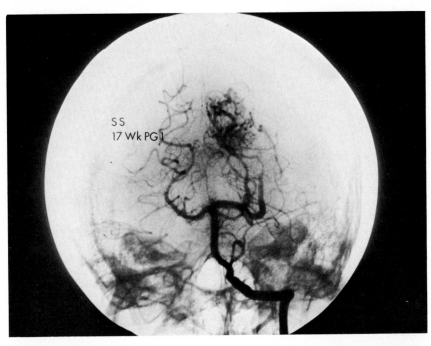

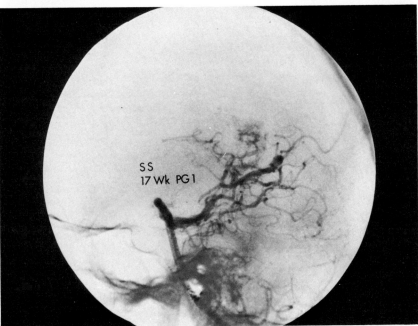

FIG. 1K (top) and **L** (bottom).   Seventeen weeks post first embolization (17 Wk PG 1) left vertebral angiogram (AP and lateral). Residual AVM.

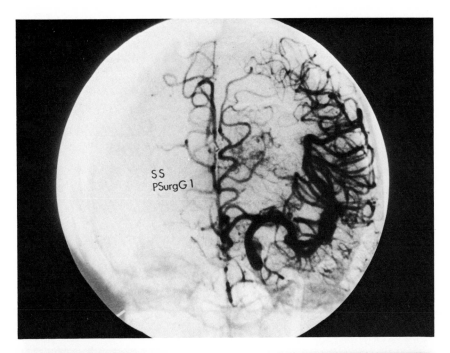

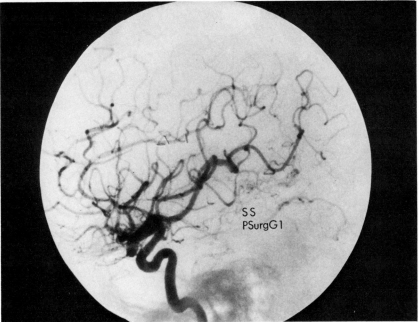

FIG. 1M (top) and **N** (bottom).   Post first intraoperative embolization (P Surg G 1) left internal carotid angiogram (AP and lateral). Minimal residual angioma visualized.

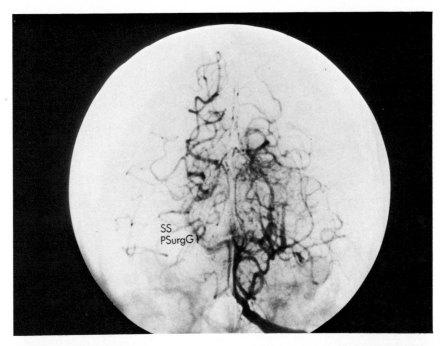

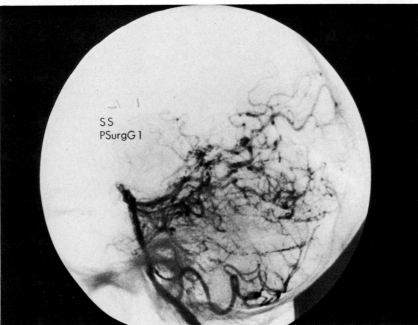

FIG. 1-O (top) and **P** (bottom).   Post first intraoperative embolization (P Surg G 1) left vertebral angiogram (AP and lateral). Minimal residual angioma.

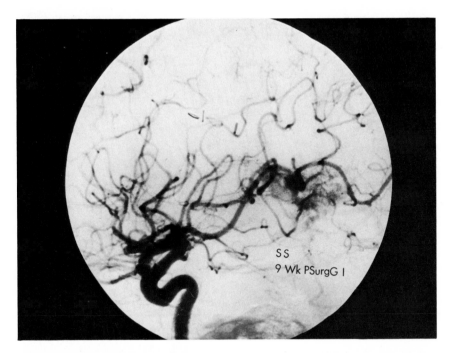

FIG. 1Q. Nine weeks post first intraoperative embolization (9 Wk P Surg G1) left internal carotid angiogram (lateral). Residual angioma demonstrated.

residual malformation fed mainly by the posterior cerebral branches with a small contribution from the middle cerebral branch. This was treated with a second mini-balloon embolization to the posterior cerebral A branches. Angiography subsequent to this procedure, immediately and 2 months later, demonstrated no evidence of residual malformation. Follow-up angiography at 6 months and yearly intervals is scheduled. His persistent mild dyslexia and mild right hemiparesis continue to improve.

Important lessons from this case are:

(a) All embolizations should be immediately followed by angiograms to demonstrate unusual or excessive vascular occlusions which may result in brain swelling sufficient to cause ventricular obstruction or mass effect.

(b) Immediate postembolization angiographic demonstration of angioma ablation (following either percutaneous mini-balloon or intraoperative embolization) is inconclusive and unreliable. Confirmation must await delayed follow-up angiography.

(c) All patients undergoing intracerebral embolization should be observed in an intensive care unit for at least 12 to 24 hr after therapy.

Case 2 (Fig. 2, A–J): A 17-year-old boy presented following hemorrhage from a dominant hemisphere deep occipital temporal AVM feeding from branches of the

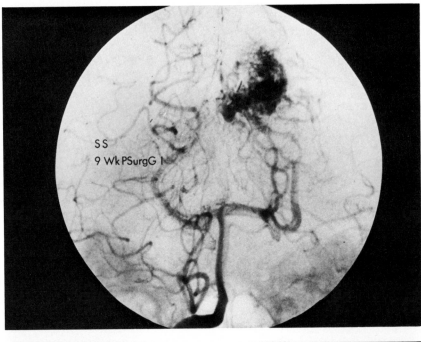

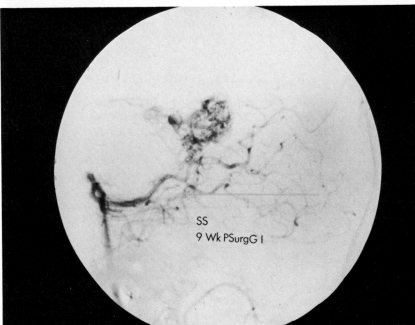

FIG. 1R (top) and **S** (bottom).   Nine weeks post first intraoperative embolization (9 Wk P Surg G 1) left vertebral angiogram (AP and lateral). Residual angioma demonstrated.

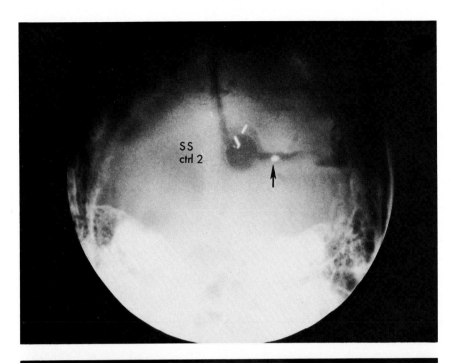

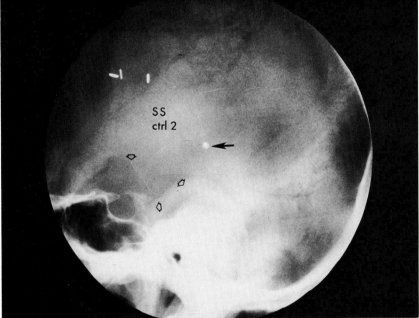

FIG. 1T (top) and **U** (bottom).   Miniature balloon position views (Ctrl 2) AP and lateral. Miniature balloon in distal left posterior cerebral artery *(arrow).*

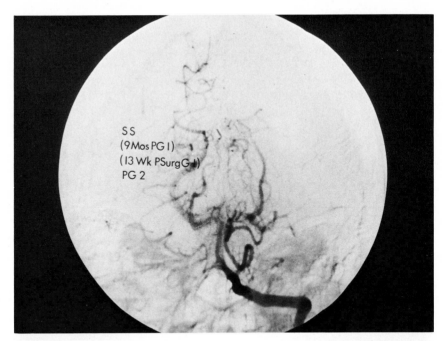

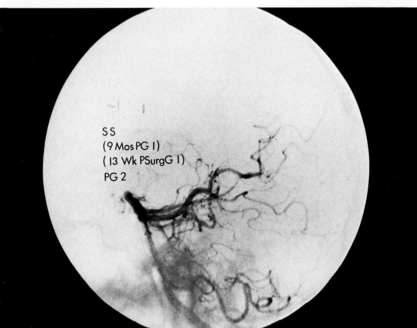

FIG. 1V (top) and **W** (bottom). Post second embolization (PG 2) left vertebral angiogram (AP and lateral). Total ablation of the angioma 9 months post first embolization and 13 weeks post first intraoperative embolization.

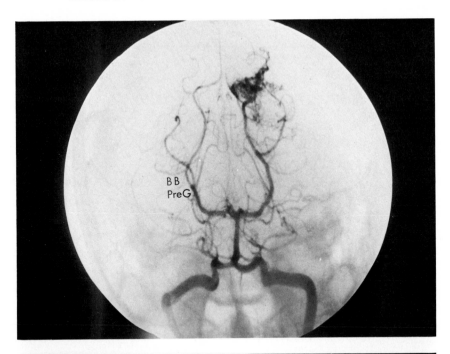

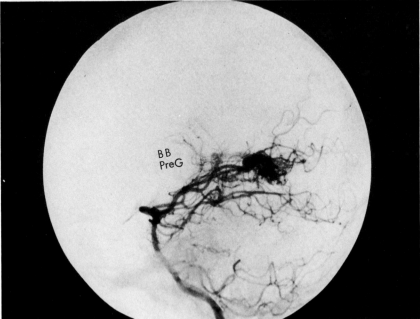

FIG. 2A (top) and **B** (bottom).   Preembolization (PreG), left vertebral angiogram (AP and lateral). Angioma fed by left posterior cerebral artery.

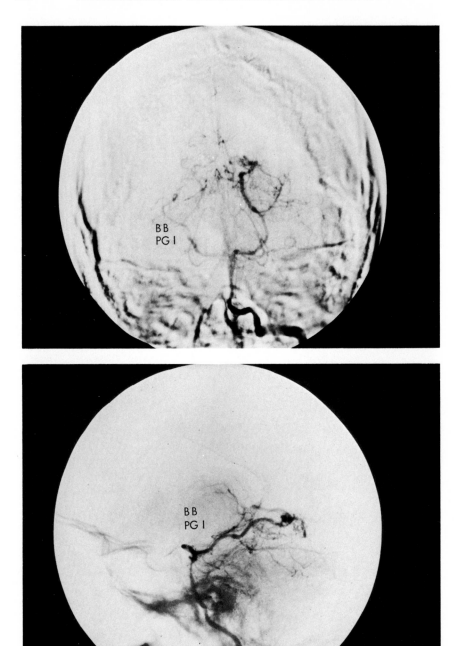

FIG. 2C (top) and **D** (bottom). Post first embolization (PG1), left vertebral angiogram (AP and lateral). Significant reduction in angioma size.

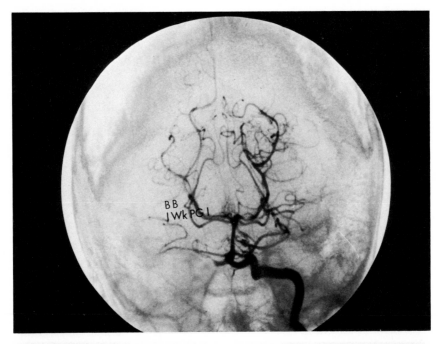

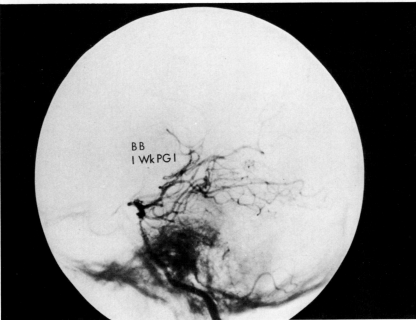

FIG. 2E (top) and **F** (bottom). One week post first embolization (PG1), left vertebral angiogram (AP and lateral). Further spontaneous reduction in angioma size.

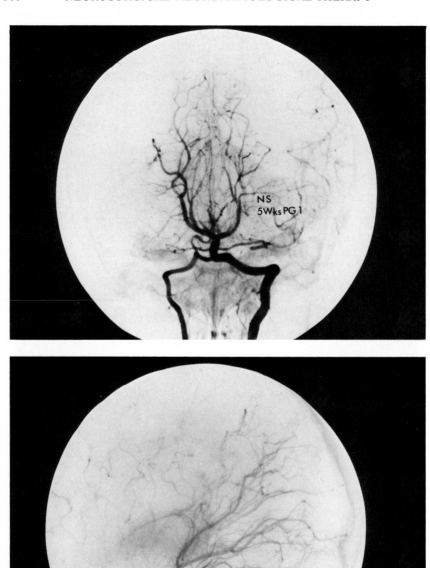

FIG. 3H   (top) and **I** (bottom). Five weeks post first embolization (5 Wks PG 1). Left vertebral angiogram (AP and lateral). Virtually complete ablation of the AVM as a result of spontaneous occlusion.

further embolization or surgery was performed and the patient will be followed with future serial angiography.

This Protocol was approved both by the Clinical Investigation and Human Use Committees at Walter Reed Army Medical Center and by the Human Use Review Office, Office of the Surgeon General (Army). The isobutyl-2-cyanoacrylate was freely supplied by Ethicon, Inc., Somerville, New Jersey, solely as a research agent. The complete protocol was approved by the Federal Food and Drug Administration (IND #G800020).

ACKNOWLEDGMENTS

We should like to acknowledge the secretarial assistance of Mrs. Elnora Barnes and Mrs. Linda Howerton and the technical assistance of Mrs. Nancy LeSueur, R. T., and Mrs. Charlene Robins, R. T.

REFERENCES

1. Banks, W. (1981): Intravascular selective occlusion. In: *Seminars on Neurological Surgery*, Raven Press, New York (*in press*).
2. Berenstein, A., and Kricheff, I. I. (1979): Catheter and material selection for transarterial embolization: Technical considerations I. *Radiology*, 132:619–631.
3. Berenstein, A., and Kricheff, I. I. (1979): Catheter and material selection for transarterial embolization: Technical considerations II. *Radiology*, 132:631–639.
4. Cromwell, L. D., and Kerber, C. W. (1979): Modification of cyanoacrylate for therapeutic embolization: Preliminary experience. *Am. J. Roentgenol.*, 132:799–801.
5. Djindjian, R. (1975): Super selective internal carotid arteriography and embolization. *Neuroradiology*, 9:145–156.
6. Doppman, J. L., Zapol, W., and Pierce, J. (1971): Transcatheter embolization with a silicone rubber preparation. Experimental observations. *Invest. Radiol.*, 6:304–309.
7. Drake, C. G. (1979): Cerebral arteriovenous malformations: Considerations for and experiences with surgical treatment in 166 cases. In: *Clinical Neurosurgery Vol. 26*, edited by Ellis B. Keener, pp. 145–208. Williams and Wilkins, Baltimore.
8. Kerber, C. W. (1975): Intracranial cyanoacrylate: A new catheter therapy for arteriovenous malformation. *Invest. Radiol.*, 10:536–538.
9. Kerber, C. W. (1976): Catheter with a calibrated leak: A new system for super selective angiography and occlusive catheter therapy. *Radiology*, 120:547–550.
10. Kunc, Z. (1974): Surgery of arteriovenous malformations in the speech and motor–sensory regions. *J. Neurosurg.*, 40:293–303.
11. Mingrino, S. (1978): Supratentorial arteriovenous malformations of the brain. *In: Advances and Technical Standards in Neurosurgery*, Vol. 5, edited by H. Krayenbuhl, et al., pp. 93–123. Springer-Verlag, Wien.
12. Pevsner, P. H. (1977): Micro-balloon catheter for super selective angiography and therapeutic occlusion. *Am. J. Roentgenol.*, 128:225–230.
13. Pevsner, P. H., and Doppman, J. L. (1980): Therapeutic embolization with a micro-balloon catheter system. *Am. J. Neuroradiol.*, 1:171–180.
14. Pevsner, P. H., and George, E. D. (1981): Therapeutic embolization of vascular lesions: Five year experience *(manuscript in preparation)*.
15. Serbinenko, F. A. (1974): Balloon catheterzation and occlusion of major cerebral vessels. *J. Neurosurg.*, 41:125–145.

Vascular Malformations, edited by
R. R. Smith, A. Haerer and W. F. Russell.
Raven Press, New York © 1982.

Aneurysms of the Great Vein of Galen: Report of Two Cases and Review of the Literature

Clinton E. Massey, Larry V. Carson, Wayne D. Beveridge, Marshall B. Allen, Jr., Betty Brooks, and F. Yaghmai

Departments of Surgery (Neurosurgery), Radiology, and Pathology, The Medical College of Georgia, Augusta, Georgia 30912

INTRODUCTION

Aneurysms of the great vein of Galen result from a fistulous connection between the arterial and venous systems deep within the posterior cranium. The clinical presentation and prognosis vary with the age of onset. Symptoms in the neonatal period primarily result from shunting of the blood and are associated with congestive heart failure. Treatment is urgent. Onset in infancy is usually associated with megalocephaly resulting from hydrocephalus. More mature children and adults usually present with headaches but may have associated hydrocephalus and intracranial calcifications. Therapy in the older age groups requires occlusion of the arteriovenous fistula and shunting of the hydrocephalus which may best be accomplished by a Torkildsen shunt.

CASE REPORTS

Case 1: DM was a 3,510-g male infant, the product of an uncomplicated pregnancy, with a history of birth asphyxia and Apgar scores of 3 and 5. Several hours following birth, the infant developed diffuse edema and anuria. Chest X-ray revealed cardiomegaly and he was referred to the Medical College of Georgia.

On arrival he was noted to be edematous. Auscultation of the heart revealed a summation gallop. The liver was palpable 6 cm below the right costal margin. The occipitofrontal circumference was 34.5 cm with an open anterior fontanelle which was pulsatile. An intracranial bruit was noted, most prominent over the left parietal area, and was synchronous with the cardiac cycle. The infant was hypotonic and unresponsive to painful stimuli.

The EKG revealed right atrial and bilateral ventricular hypertrophy. Chest X-ray showed massive cardiac enlargement. An unenhanced CT scan showed a high-density mass just to the left of the midline with an interhemispheric area of increased density believed to represent a dilated vein of Galen and straight sinus (Fig. 1).

The infant was started on digoxin without benefit. Diuretics failed to produce

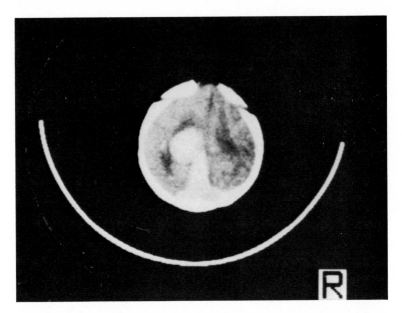

FIG. 1. Case 1. Unenhanced CT scan showing areas of high attenuation in the regions of the vein of Galen and straight sinus.

improvement in renal status. A cerebral angiogram was attempted through an umbilical artery approach but was terminated prior to injection because of ventricular fibrillation.

The infant was resuscitated but died at 6 days of age in congestive heart failure without evidence of brainstem function. A postmortem intracardiac angiogram revealed an arteriovenous malformation (AVM) of the cerebral vessels with dilatation of the venous dural sinuses, including the vein of Galen (Fig. 2). Examination of the brain demonstrated infarction and atrophy of both cerebral hemispheres. With the exception of hypertrophy, the heart was normal.

Case 2: LB is a 36-year-old white male, first seen at the Medical College of Georgia on January 2, 1980 because of a recent decrease in his productivity at a workshop for the mentally retarded. He gave a history of a large head since infancy for which medical advice was never sought, and occasional frontal and occipital headaches lasting for 2 to 3 days at a time, unrelieved by aspirin or Tylenol. He also reported a recent decrease in his visual acuity. Past medical history revealed previous treatment for systemic arterial hypertension.

The patient presented as a thin male with macrocephaly, the occipitofrontal circumference measuring 68 cm. Dilated veins were present in the glabellar region bilaterally. The remainder of the patient's general physical examination was unremarkable with the exception of a blood pressure of 156/96 supine. Neurological examination revealed a cooperative male who was alert and oriented. He expressed

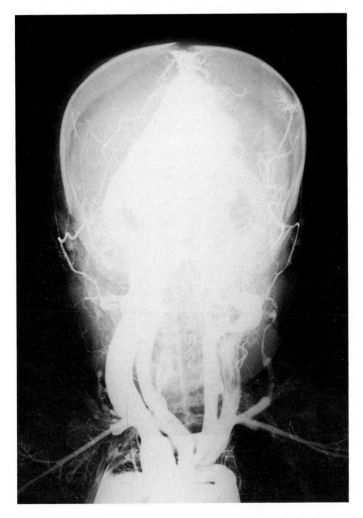

FIG. 2. Case 1. Frontal **(A)** and lateral **(B)** views of the postmortem angiogram showing a dilated vein of Galen and straight sinus, as well as the deep cerebral vermiform mass of vessels.

concern about his head size, stating that he was "funny-looking." His judgment and insight were believed to be consistent with mild retardation. He had an intention tremor bilaterally, greater in the left upper extremity. Rapid alternating movements and finger tapping abilities were impaired bilaterally. The sensory examination was normal. His Romberg was negative. He had moderately increased muscle tone to passive motion throughout. No pathological reflexes were elicited.

Skull X-rays revealed two calcified masses in the midline (Fig. 3). One of these masses was in the region of the pineal and the other in the area of the torcula. A

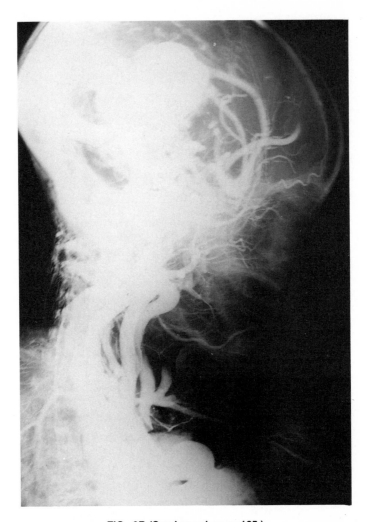

FIG. 2B.(See legend on p. 165.)

CT scan showed the lesion in the region of the pineal to be cystic and filled with a material of high density. There was further enhancement after intravenous injection of contrast medium. The lateral and third ventricles were markedly dilated (Fig. 4). The findings were believed to be consistent with an aneurysm of the great vein of Galen and obstructive hydrocephalus. A radionuclide brain scan demonstrated patency of the aneurysm. A four-vessel cerebral angiogram confirmed the diagnosis. The aneurysm was fed by branches of the right posterior cerebral artery, which filled from both the anterior and posterior intracranial circulation (Fig. 5). The EEG

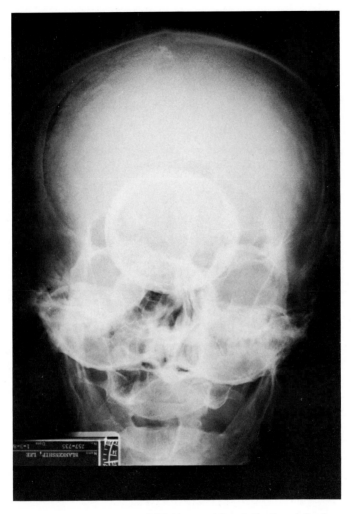

FIG. 3. Case 2. Frontal **(A)** and lateral **(B)** X-rays of the skull with calcifications present in the region of the pineal and torcula. (Courtesy of The Williams and Wilkins Company, Baltimore, MD.)

was normal. An ophthalmological consultant found a refractory error only. Neuropsychological evaluation revealed a Wechsler IQ of 62.

The patient underwent a ventriculoperitoneal shunt using a medium pressure valve for treatment of his hydrocephalus. His postoperative course was unventful; however, the patient did appear somewhat emotionally depressed, and following the recommendation of a psychiatric consultant, he was placed on Elavil. The

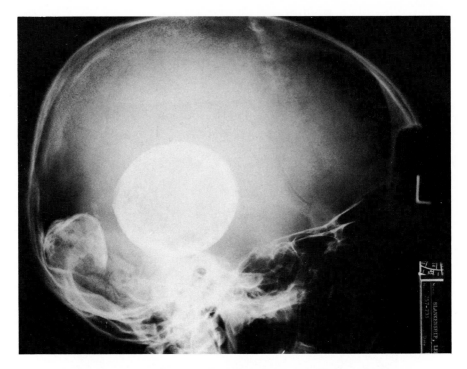

FIG. 3B. (See legend on p. 167.)

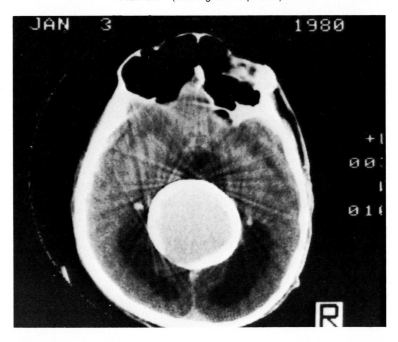

FIG. 4. Case 2. Enhanced CT scan revealing the dilated vein of Galen with its calcified wall and enhancing contents.

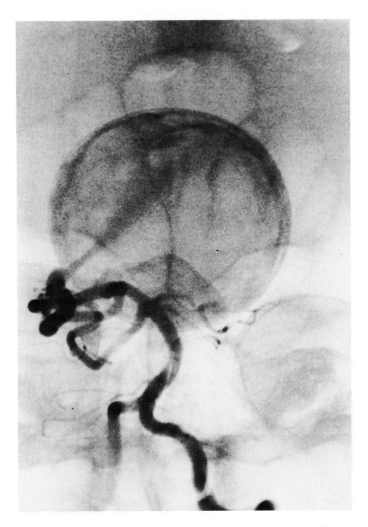

FIG. 5. Case 2. Subtracted views of the magnified vertebral angiogram, **(A)** frontal and **(B)** lateral, showing a jet of contrast material entering the vein of Galen through a dilated right posterior cerebral artery. (Courtesy of The Williams and Wilkins Company, Baltimore, MD).

patient was discharged from the hospital with relief of his headaches. His neurological examination was unchanged from that on admission.

Approximately 6 weeks following his discharge the patient was readmitted obtunded and with cellulitis of his right ear. Three weeks earlier he had fallen, following which he had been admitted to a local hospital with a decreased level of consciousness and an abrasion to his right ear. At the time of his second admission a CT scan revealed bilateral subdural effusions. These were drained and his ventriculoperitoneal shunt was ligated. Postoperatively his level of consciousness improved; however, he began to complain of recurrent headaches. He was therefore

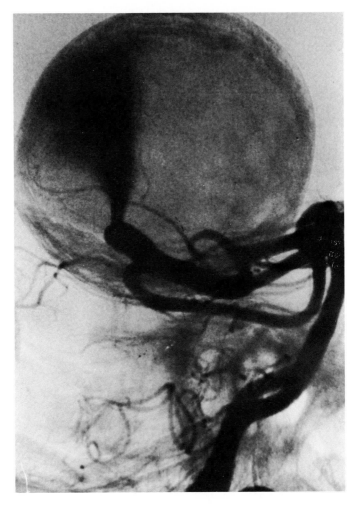

FIG. 5B.

returned to the operating room and his ventriculoperitioneal shunt reestablished with the substitution of a high pressure valve. Follow-up CT scan, 2 days later, revealed reaccumulation of his subdural effusions. Subsequently, through an interhemispheric approach, the feeding vessels to the dilated vein of Galen were clipped and his shunt ligated .He subsequently did well and was discharged from the hospital.

    LB was admitted to the hospital for the third time 4 months later because of recurrent headaches. Repeat angiography revealed occlusion of the feeding vessels to the aneurysm (Fig. 6). Because of his continued complaints of headaches, a Torkildsen shunt was performed during this admission.

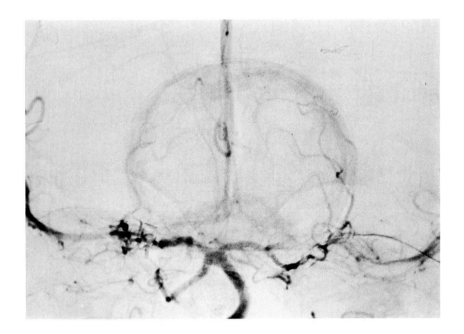

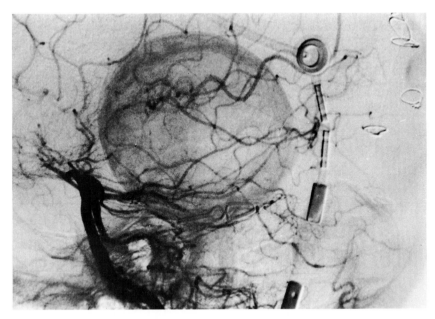

FIG. 6A. (top) and **B** (bottom). **Case 2.**   Postoperative subtracted vertebral angiogram in the magnified frontal **(A)** and lateral **(B)** projections, showing occlusion of the fistula and the position of the Drake aneurysm clip on branches of the posterior cerebral artery. (Courtesy of The Williams and Wilkins Company, Baltimore, MD).

He has done well since. His ventricles have not decreased in size and complaints of headaches are rare. Repeat neuropsychological testing demonstrated that his IQ remains below the fifth percentile at approximately 70. Six months following the occlusion of the vessels feeding his aneurysm, he has returned to work and is asymptomatic except for occasional headaches.

DISCUSSION

Although Dandy (14) attributes the first reported case of arteriovenous aneurysm of the brain to Steinheil in 1895, the first definitive aneurysm of the vein of Galen was not reported until 1937 when Jaeger et al. (25,26) reported a case of "bilateral congenital cerebral arteriovenous communication." Since that time there have been some 80 such aneurysms reported in the English literature (1–4,6,7,9–13,15–24,27,28,30–36,38,39,41–45,47–53), Case 2 reported here having been previously reported by Carson et al. (11).

The term "aneurysm of the vein of Galen" is in reality a misnomer. A more proper description would be arteriovenous fistula with distention of the vein of Galen. Many authors (6,7,14,19,26,32,36,37,40,46) have addressed the classification of AVMs of the brain. Litvak et al. (32) specifically address the issue of "midline arteriovenous anomalies" and classify such anomalies into three categories; (a) aneurysm of the great vein of Galen, (b) racemose conglomerations draining into the great vein or other deep venous channels, and (c) transitional lesions in which there is a direct anomalous connection between the arteries and veins other than the great vein or drainage of the "angiomas" to structures other than the deep cerebral veins, i.e., directly into the dural sinuses. Gold et al. (19) emphasize that, in the "classic" aneurysm of the vein of Galen, the fistulous connection is direct without an interposed "angioma." The second case of this report illustrates this concept well. Case 1, on the other hand, is an example of a large AVM which ultimately drains via the great cerebral vein causing dilatation of the vein and dural sinuses. In both cases the aneurysmal dilatation of the vein of Galen is secondary to the vascular shunt and not a "true" aneurysm.

Forty-nine of the 72 cases reported in which the sex was given were males (Table 1). About three quarters of the reported patients became symptomatic prior to the second year of life. Cohen et al. (13), reporting the occurrence in a 52-year-old male, emphasized that this lesion is not restricted to infants or children.

TABLE 1. *Sex distribution*

Total cases:	72
Males	49
Females	23
Ratio	2:1

SIGNS AND SYMPTOMS

Patients harboring aneurysms of the great vein of Galen present with one or more of three symptom complexes: (a) congestive heart failure, (b) hydrocephalus, or (c) headaches. Gold et al. (19) in 1964 and Amacher and Shillito (4) in 1973 extensively reviewed the literature on aneurysms of the great vein of Galen and found that the clinical presentation correlated well with the age at which the patient developed symptoms. Gold et al. (19) divided the cases into three age groups: (a) neonatal, (b) infancy, (c) older children and adults. This classification, as defined by us, is shown in Table 2. Neonates presented with congestive heart failure. Older infants had hydrocephalus, and headache was the most frequent complaint of those patients who initially presented as older children or adults. Amacher and Shillito (4) described a fourth category: infants, who had mild congestive heart failure as neonates, but who later developed hydrocephalus.

Table 3 relates the most common findings in patients with an aneurysm of the great vein of Galen to the age of presentation. Satisfactory information is available in only 70 patients obtained from the literature.

Ninety-five percent of the patients who became symptomatic prior to 1 month of age showed evidence of severe congestive heart failure. In all cases the failure was resistant to digitalization. Many of these children were referred for evaluation

TABLE 2. *Classification according to age*

Neonates
Less than 1 month of age
Infants
1 to 24 months of age
Older children and adults
Greater than 24 months of age

TABLE 3. *Clinical findings with respect to age of patient*

Clinical feature	Neonates		Infants		Children and adults	
	No.	%	No.	%	No.	%
Congestive heart failure	20	95	10	29	1	7
Hydrocephalus	0	0	28	82	5	36
Headache	0	0	0	0	10	71
Seizures	4	19	7	20	1	7
Calcification on skull X-ray	0	0	1	3	10	71
Intracranial bruit	8	38	13	37	2	14
Subarachnoid hemorrhage	1	5	2	6	5	36
Total patients	21		35		14	

of congenital heart disease. An occasional patient who presented later than 1 month of age had evidence of congestive heart failure. The failure in these infants was usually mild and responded to digitalization. Some had only radiographic and/or electrocardiographic evidence of heart failure (i.e., enlarged cardiac silhouette or axis deviation). Levine et al. (31) concluded that the time of appearance of the cardiac decompensation depends primarily on the size of the shunt and that lowering of the peripheral vascular resistance was the etiology of the clinical and hemodynamic changes. The lowered peripheral resistance leads to a compensatory increase in blood volume and cardiac output in order to maintain perfusion of the systemic vascular bed. Glatt and Rowe (18) recommended consideration of an arteriovenous fistula in infants with congestive heart failure that is refractory to digitalization if congenital heart disease has been excluded. The presence of a bruit over the skull makes the diagnosis of a cerebral arteriovenous fistula likely and cerebral angiography is imperative.

Eighty percent of individuals who have arteriovenous fistulae involving the great vein of Galen were found to have an increased head circumference if they did not develop refractory congestive heart failure during the first month of life. Bedford (8), after a series of studies in dogs in which ligation of the vein of Galen failed to produce hydrocephalus, concluded that the hydrocephalus was secondary to compression of the midbrain. Disturbance of cerebrospinal fluid absorption could contribute to the development of hydrocephalus if subarachnoid hemorrhage has occurred (5).

Seventy-one percent of patients initially evaluated as children or adults for aneurysms of the great vein of Galen complained of headaches of variable duration. The presence of hydrocephalus in the adult group presents a treatment dilemma, especially if the hydrocephalus is long standing and massive, as in Case 2 presented here. Standard ventriculoperitoneal shunts are complicated by bilateral subdural hematomas in these patients. A Torkildsen shunt may allow for adequate release of the intracranial pressure without the risk of rapid ventricular decompression as is the case with the ventriculoperitoneal shunt.

Thirty-six percent of the adult patients have evidence of at least one subarachnoid hemorrhage. The exact incidence of subarachnoid hemorrhage is not known but Cohen et al. (13) made the observation that patients with deep AVMs appeared to have a lower incidence of hemorrhage than those with cortically placed malformations. Hirano and Solomon (22) reported a case of an aneurysm of the great vein of Galen in which the patient suffered a subarachnoid hemorrhage. At postmortem examination the source of bleeding was identified as a distal vein, not the aneurysmally dilated vein of Galen. It may be that these patients have a high risk of subarachnoid hemorrhage from dilated veins but that rupture of the aneurysmally dilated vein of Galen itself is unlikely.

RADIOGRAPHIC ASPECTS

Curvilinear calcifications are seen frequently on the plain skull X-rays of patients over 15 years of age. One infant reported by Weir et al. (49) with such calcification at 7 months of age was subsequently found to have a completely thrombosed aneurysm. Wilson and Roy (50) state that concentric calcification on skull X-rays is pathognomonic for aneurysms of the vein of Galen if the following three criteria are met: (a) the deposits are thin and delicate and form a complete or incomplete ring, (b) they are located in the region of the pineal, and (c) they measure greater than 2.5 cm in diameter.

Cerebral angiography is now the definitive diagnostic procedure. Boldrey and Miller (10) in 1949 reported the first case diagnosed preoperatively by angiography. Table 4 lists the feeding vessels in 53 patients. The posterior cerebral arteries were involved in approximately 87% of the cases and provided the sole supply to the aneurysm in about 50%. The right posterior cerebral artery was more often involved than the left.

TREATMENT

Obliteration of the arteriovenous fistula should be the treatment of choice. Talalla (45) has stated that clipping of the feeding vessels is sufficient. Amacher and Shillito (4) apparently agree. In their report of five surgical cases, they did not attempt excision or plication of the sac. A right occipital craniotomy as described by Lazar and Clark (29), and utilized in approaching the aneurysm in the present report allows adequate exposure of the region and also access to the ventricular system for tapping if necessary.

TABLE 4. *Arterial feeders (N = 52)*

Artery	Involved	Only supply
Posterior cerebral		
Bilateral	22	11
Right	17	11
Left	8	4
Anterior cerebral		
Bilateral	2	0
Right	2	0
Left	3	0
Middle cerebral		
Bilateral	1	0
Right	1	0
Left	2	0
Anterior choroidal		
Bilateral	1	0
Right	1	0
Left	1	1
Superior cerebellar	4	1
Posterior communicating		
Bilateral	1	1
Right	3	0
Left	1	0
Pericallosal	2	0
Vertebral	1	0
Right occipital	1	0

TABLE 5. *Treatment (N = 70)*

Group	Total patients		Operated patients		Postop survivors		Unoperated survivors		Total survivors	
	No.	%	No.	%	No.	%	No.	%	No.	%
Neonatal	21	100	6	29	2	33	0	0	2	10
Infants	34	100	25	74	15	60	1	3	16	47
Children and adults	16	100	11	69	8	73	1	6	9	56

Table 5 gives the surgical experience as reported in the literature. Of 21 neonatal cases only 6 have undergone attempted surgical correction of the fistula prior to 1 month of age, with only two survivors. The first reported successful ligation was by Gomez et al. (20) in 1963. The neonate underwent ligation of the right common carotid and left external carotid arteries with resultant disappearance of the intracranial bruit and resolution of the congestive heart failure. Amacher and Shillito (4) reported the second case of successful surgical treatment in a neonate with mild congestive heart failure who underwent intracranial ligation of the fistula. Interestingly, several of the neonates with severe congestive heart failure who have undergone surgical obliteration of the arteriovenous fistula had persistent postoperative cardiac decompensation which remained resistant to digitalization and phlebotomy. Although the pathophysiology underlying this situation is poorly understood it may be that, since the heart is normally working at near maximum ability in the neonate, the added stress created by the arteriovenous shunt may produce sufficient myocardial damage to prevent recovery following closure of the shunt. Following closure of the arteriovenous fistula the peripheral vascular resistance increases markedly as noted by Levine et al. (31), with resultant continued stress on the left side of the heart. The persistence of postoperative cardiac failure may be minimized with careful phlebotomy and restriction of intraoperative and postoperative fluids.

Clearly the prognosis for patients with arteriovenous fistulae of the vein of Galen who present in the neonatal period is dismal. However, it must be recognized that in spite of the poor outlook, the only reasonable chance of survival for these infants is surgical occlusion of the fistula. Therefore patients who present with clinical evidence suggestive of an arteriovenous fistula (severe congestive heart failure and intracranial bruit) represent a neurosurgical emergency and cerebral angiography should be performed on an urgent basis. If the angiogram demonstrates direct arterial communication, surgical occlusion of the fistula should be attempted with the realization that even with surgical correction the outlook is poor. The angiogram may reveal a more complex vascular anomaly, as in the first case, which may not be as amenable to surgical treatment.

The prognosis for older patients is better (Table 5). Approximately 50% of infants and older persons survive.

SUMMARY

Aneurysms of the vein of Galen have been verified in 80 cases recovered from the English literature, including the cases herein reported. There is a marked male predominance in these cases.

The patients can be conveniently divided into three groups based on age and presenting clinical picture. The youngest symptomatic patients are the neonates who present with congestive heart failure secondary to the arteriovenous shunt. The second group is comprised of infants between 1 and 24 months of age who generally present with hydrocephalus secondary to occlusion of the aqueduct of Sylvius by the dilated vein of Galen. A third group of patients made up of young children and adults generally present with headaches. The presence of curvilinear calcifications seen in the area of the pineal on plain skull X-rays is usual in this older group.

The cerebral angiogram, including both anterior and posterior circulation, is the definitive diagnostic procedure. In a review of the literature, the posterior cerebral artery is most commonly involved, providing the sole supply in 50% of the cases.

The outlook for those patients presenting prior to 1 month of age is dismal with only two survivors among the 21 cases reported, one of whom had very mild heart failure. These patients are believed to represent a neurosurgical emergency in that obliteration of the fistula provides the only chance for survival, albeit poor. The outlook for the second and third groups is better.

In general, occlusion of the fistula is the first treatment required, followed by control of hydrocephalus as indicated. In the adult patients, with massive hydrocephalus and fixed skulls, a Torkildsen shunt may be the method of choice for shunting, since there appears to be a lesser likelihood of postshunt subdural hematomas.

REFERENCES

1. Agee, O. F., and Greer, M. (1967); Anomalous cephalic venous drainage in association with aneurysm of the great vein of Galen. *Radiology*, 88:725–729.
2. Agee, O. F., Musella, R., and Tweed, C. G. (1969): Aneurysm of the great vein of Galen: Report of two cases. *J. Neurosurg.*, 31:346–351.
3. Alpers, B. J., and Forster, F. M. (1945): Arteriovenous aneurysm of great cerebral vein and arteries of Circle of Willis. *Arch. Neurol. Psychiatry*, 54:181–185.
4. Amacher, A. L., and Shillito, J. (1973): The syndromes and surgical treatment of aneurysms of the great vein of Galen. *J. Neurosurg.*, 39:89–98.
5. Askenasy, H. M., Herzberger, E. E., and Wigenbeck, H. S. (1953): Hydrocephalus with vascular malformation of the brain: A preliminary report. *Neurology (Minneap.)*, 3:213–220.
6. Aube, M., Tenner, M. S., Brown, J., and Sher, J. (1975): Arteriovenous malformation of the vein of Galen. *Acta Radiol. Suppl.*, 347:23–30.
7. Bartal, A. D. (1975): Classification of aneurysm of the great vein of Galen (Letter to the Editor). *J. Neurosurg.*, 42:617–619.
8. Bedford, T. H. B.(1934): The great vein of Galen and the syndrome of increased intracranial pressure. *Brain*, 57:1–24.
9. Berger, P. E., Harwood-Nash, D. C., and Fitz, C. R. (1976): Computerized tomography: Abnormal intracerebral collections of blood in children. *Neuroradiology*, 11:29–33.
10. Boldrey, E., and Miller, E. R. (1949): Arteriovenous fistula (aneurysm) of the great cerebral vein (of Galen) and the Circle of Willis. *Arch. Neurol. Psychiatry*, 62:778–783.

11. Carson, L. V., Brooks, B. S., ElGammal, T., Massey, C. E., Beveridge, W. D., and Allen, M. B., Jr. (1981): Adult arteriovenous malformation of the vein of Galen: A case report with pre- and postoperative CT findings. *Neurosurgery*, 7:495–498.
12. Claireaux, A. E., and Newman, C. G. H. (1960): Arteriovenous aneurysm of the great vein of Galen with heart failure in the neonatal period. *Arch. Dis. Child.*, 35:605–612.
13. Cohen, M. M., Kristiansen, K., and Hval, E. (1954): Arteriovenous malformations of the great vein of Galen. *Neurology (Minneap.)*, 4:124–127.
14. Dandy, W. E. (1928): Arteriovenous aneurysm of the brain. *Arch. Surg.*, 17:190–243.
15. French, L. A., and Peyton, W. T. (1954): Vascular malformations in the region of the great vein of Galen. *J. Neurosurg.*, 11:488–498.
16. Gagnon, J., and Boileau, G. (1960): Anatomical study of an arteriovenous malformation drained by the system of Galen. *J. Neurosurg.*, 17:75–80.
17. Gibson, J. B., Taylor, A. R., and Richardson, A. E. (1959): Congenital arteriovenous fistula with an aneurysm of the great cerebral vein and hydrocephalus treated surgically. *J. Neurol. Neurosurg. Psychiatry*, 22:224–228.
18. Glatt, B. S., and Rowe, R. D. (1960): Cerebral arteriovenous fistula associated with congestive heart failure in the newborn; Report of two cases. *Pediatrics*, 26:596–603.
19. Gold, A. P., Ransohoff, J., and Carter, S. (1964): Vein of Galen malformation. *Acta Neurol. Scand. [Suppl. 11]*, 40:5–31.
20. Gomez, M. R., Whitten, C. F., Nolke, A., Bernstein, J., and Meyer, J. S. (1963): Aneurysmal malformation of the great vein of Galen causing heart failure in early infancy. *Pediatrics*, 31:400–411.
21. Heinz, E. R., Schwartz, J. F., and Sears, R. A. (1968): Thrombosis in the vein of Galen malformations. *Br. J. Radiol.*, 41:424–428.
22. Hirano, A., and Solomon, S. (1960): Arteriovenous aneurysm of the vein of Galen. *Arch. Neurol.*, 5:589–593.
23. Hirano, A., and Terry, R. D. (1958): Aneurysm of the vein of Galen. *J. Neuropathol. Exp. Neurol.*, 17:424–429.
24. Hood, J. B., Wallace, C. T., and Mahaffey, J. E. (1977): Anesthetic management of an intracranial arteriovenous malformation in infancy. *Anesth. Analg.*, 56:236–241.
25. Jaeger, J. R., Forbes, R. P., and Dandy, W. E. (1937): Bilateral congenital cerebral arteriovenous communication aneurysm. *Trans. Am. Neurol. Assoc.*, 173–176.
26. Jaeger, J. R., and Forbes, R. P. (1946): Bilateral congenital arteriovenous communications (aneurysm) of the cerebral vessels. *Arch. Neurol. Psychiatry*, 55:591–599.
27. Kalyanaraman, K., Jagannathan, K., and Ramamurthi, B. (1971): Vein of Galen malformation with atypical manifestations: A case report. *Dev. Med. Child Neurol.*, 13:625–629.
28. Lazar, M. L. (1974): Vein of Galen aneurysm: Successful excision of a completely thrombosed aneurysm in an infant. *Surg. Neurol.*, 2:22–24.
29. Lazar, M. L., and Clark, K. (1974): Direct surgical management of masses in the region of the vein of Galen. *Surg. Neurol.*, 2:17–21.
30. Lehman, J. S., Chynn, K. Y., Hagstrom, J. W. C., and Steinberg, I. (1966): Heart failure in infancy due to arteriovenous malformations of the vein of Galen. *Am. J. Roentgenol.*, 98:653–659.
31. Levine, O. R., Jameson, A. G., Nellhaus, G., and Gold, A. P. (1962): Cardiac complications of cerebral arteriovenous fistula in infancy. *Pediatrics*, 30:563–575.
32. Litvak, J., Yahr, M. D., and Ransohoff, J. (1960): Aneurysms of the great vein of Galen and midline cerebral arteriovenous anomalies. *J. Neurosurg.*, 17:945–954.
33. Lumsden, C. E. (1947): A case of aneurysm of the vein of Galen. *J. Pathol. Bacteriol.*, 59:328–331.
34. Morris, L. (1971): Pneumoencephalographic findings in a case of vein of Galen aneurysm. *Br. J. Radiol.*, 44:798–801.
35. Norman, M. G., and Becker, L. E. (1974): Cerebral damage in neonates resulting from arteriovenous malformation of the vein of Galen. *J. Neurol. Neurosurg. Psychiatry*, 37:252–258.
36. O'Brien, M. S., and Schechter, M. D. (1970): Arteriovenous malformations involving the Galenic system. *Am. J. Roentgenol.*, 110:50–55.
37. Olivecrona, H., and Riives, J. (1948): Arteriovenous aneurysms of the brain. *Arch. Neurol. Psychiatry*, 59:567–602.
38. Oscherwitz, D., and Davidoff, L. M. (1947): Midline calcified intracranial aneurysms between occipital lobes. *J. Neurosurg.*, 4:539–541.

39. Poppen, J. L., and Avman, N. (1960): Aneurysms of the great vein of Galen. *J. Neurosurg.*, 17:238–244.
40. Ray, B. S. (1941): Cerebral arteriovenous aneurysms. *Surg. Gynecol. Obstet.*, 73:615–648.
41. Russell, D. S., and Nevin, S. (1940): Aneurysm of the great vein of Galen, causing internal hydrocephalus: Report of two cases. *J. Pathol. Bacteriol.*, 51:375–383.
42. Russell, W., and Newton, T. H. (1964): Aneurysm of the vein of Galen. *Am. J. Roentgenol.*, 92:756–760.
43. Siqueira, E. B., and Murray, K. J. (1972): Calcified aneurysms of the vein of Galen: Report of a presumed case and review of the literature. *Neurochirurgia*, 3:106–112.
44. Stehbens, W. E., Sahgal, K. K., Nelson, L., and Shaher, R. M. (1973): Aneurysm of vein of Galen and diffuse meningeal angiectasia. *Arch. Pathol.*, 95:333–335.
45. Talalla, A. (1973): Vein of Galen aneurysm. *Bull. Los Angeles Neurol. Soc.*, 38:110–121.
46. Thompson, J. R., Harwood-Nash, D. C., and Fitz, C. R. (1973): Cerebral aneurysms in children. *Am. J. Roentgenol.*, 118:163–175.
47. Thomson, J. L. G. (1959): Aneurysm of the vein of Galen. *Br. J. Radiol.*, 32:680–684.
48. Verdura, J., and Shafron, M. (1969): Aneurysm of vein of Galen in infancy. *Surgery*, 65:494–498.
49. Weir, B. K. A., Allen, P. B. R., and Miller, J. D. R. (1968): Excision of thrombosed vein of Galen aneurysm in an infant. *J. Neurosurg.*, 29:619–622.
50. Wilson, C. B., and Roy, M. (1964): Calcification within congenital aneurysms of the vein of Galen. *Am. J. Roentgenol.*, 91:1319–1326.
51. Wolfe, H. R. I., and France, N. E. (1949): Arteriovenous aneurysms of the great vein of Galen. *Br. J. Surg.*, 37:76–78.
52. Young, L. W. (1977): Radiological case of the month. *Am. J. Dis. Child.*, 131:581–582.
53. Zingessar, L. H., Schechter, M. M., Kier, E. L., and O'Brien, M. S. (1969): Vascular malformations of the posterior fossa including the tentorial hiatus. *Am. J. Roentgenol.*, 105:341–347.

Vascular Malformations, edited by
R. R. Smith, A. Haerer and W. F. Russell.
Raven Press, New York © 1982.

Neuro-Ophthalmological Aspects of Carotid Cavernous Fistula

Larry Parker

*Division of Neuro-Ophthalmology, University of Mississippi Medical Center,
Jackson, Mississippi 39216*

Carotid cavernous fistulas (CCF) have an approximate incidence of 1 per 10,000 to 1 per 20,000 hospital admissions. An anatomically unique arrangement of the vascular system predisposes the formation of such a fistula. A major artery, the carotid, directly passes through a plexiform dural venous sinus, the cavernous sinus. Any circumstance that violates the integrity of the cavernous carotid arterial wall will therefore lead to direct fistulous connection between a major artery and a large venous sinus. Only in the sphenoparietal and petrosal sinuses is this vascular arrangement partially duplicated, as small penetrating arteries are found coursing through these dural venous channels (20). Trauma is the etiology in 75% of CCFs. An opening in the intracavernous carotid artery is created by blunt, penetrating, or iatrogenic surgically induced orbitocranial injuries (10,18). Twenty-five percent of CCFs are "spontaneous," with no prior history of trauma. Large or small intracavernous arteries may communicate with the cavernous sinus via aneurysmal rupture, or through defects in the arterial wall caused by inherited connective tissue diseases or advanced arteriosclerosis (3,6,14). Dural arterial-venous shunts may also produce a symptomatic "spontaneous" CCF when branches of the external or internal carotid artery communicate with dural veins in the vicinity of the cavernous sinus (12).

In either etiological category, arterialized blood empties directly into the cavernous sinus and then must egress this sinus via several paths (Fig. 1A.) These exit channels are most important, since clinical symptomatology will largely be determined by the specific engorged, arterialized veins, which carry the major portion of the fistulous blood flow away from the cavernous sinus. The largest and most frequently utilized pathway is flow in an anterior direction out of the cavernous sinus into the superior and inferior ophthalmic veins. The superior ophthalmic vein in particular may become immensely enlarged (Fig. 1A), and may be easily seen on contrasted computerized tomographic (CT) scans (Fig. 1B). Ipsilateral neuro-ophthalmological symptoms are thus produced from the ensuing orbital and ocular venous enlargement and congestion. Intracavernous venous connections are also present which may carry a significant amount of blood into the opposite cavernous sinus. If egress of blood from the fellow cavernous sinus is then accomplished via anterior ophthalmic venous channels, asymmetrical bilateral, or predominantly contralateral neuro-ophthalmological symptoms occur (4). If blood exits the cavernous sinus primarily via lateral, posterior, or inferior venous drainage routes, traditional

TABLE 1. *Neuroophthalmological signs and symptoms in carotid cavernous fistula*

Bruit
Exophthalmos
Pulsation
Conjunctival involvement and chemosis
Lid and facial skin changes
Cranial nerve involvement
Headache
Glaucoma
Miscellaneous ocular findings
   Corneal involvement—exposure; haze or edema
   Anterior chamber—cell and flare; neovascularization of
     the angle; glaucoma
   Iris—pupillary paralysis, iris atrophy; posterior synechiae
   Lens—cataract
   Retina—venous engorgement; venous stasis retinopathy;
     detachment
   Optic disk—edema; optic atrophy; ischemic optic neuropathy;
     neovascularization; glaucomatous cupping

---

both to orbital congestion and edema, and increased size of the ophthalmic veins. The superior ophthalmic vein often drains prominently into the angular vein, situated in the superiomedial portion of the anterior orbit. For this reason the eye is frequently displaced anteriorly, laterally, and downward (Fig. 2). Exophthalmometer readings disclose from 2 to 20 mm of proptosis, with an average of 8 to 10 mm (19). Pulsation of the exophthalmos is a variable sign reported in 27% of Henderson's series, and in 80% of Martin and Mabon's series (8,11). The pulsation results from transmission of an arterial pulse wave down the superior ophthalmic vein into the orbit. It can be detected by viewing the eye from the side, observing pulsatile movements of a finger placed over the eye, or by viewing the eye with an exophthalmometer. Boyes and Ralph (2) described a "swinging tonometer sign," which may be present in the absence of visible ocular pulsation. While measuring intraocular pressure with a Schiotz tonometer, they noted a 6 to 8 division swing of the tonometer, synchronous with the patient's pulse. No visible pulsation by inspection was observable in their patient.

Chemosis refers to the hyperemia, engorgement, and increase in size of the bulbar and palpebral conjunctiva, seen in some patients with CCF. Conjunctival involvement varies in reported series from 36 to 79% (7,15). Chemosis is often most marked acutely after the onset of a traumatic fistula. When pronounced, it is frequently worse inferiorly, with the inferior bulbar and palpebral conjunctiva at times prolapsing through the palpebral fissure (Fig. 3). The prolapsed conjunctiva may then dry out, ulcerate, necrose, bleed freely, or become infected. With improved orbital anastomotic outflow, chemosis improves, and is replaced by dilated, thickened, arterialized conjunctival and episcleral vessels (Fig. 3). These vessels are larger and more tortuous than inflammatory vessels. They also frequently extend from the periphery to the limbus, whereas inflammatory episcleral vessels most often leave a perilimbal clear zone. If severed, these veins may bleed profusely, and hemostasis is occasionally alarmingly difficult to achieve. Other lid and facial

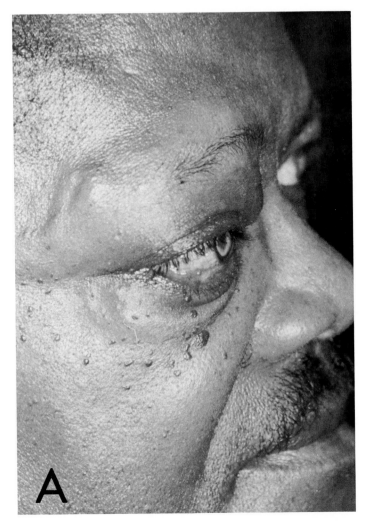

FIG. 2A. Exophthalmos as viewed from the side. Also seen are the lid and facial enlargements caused by dilated veins.

changes include chronic, grotesque, vermiform subcutaneous enlargements. The angular and facial veins particularly enlarge to carry blood from the ophthalmic veins to the jugular venous system. These enlargements are most frequently and uniformly seen superomedially in the orbit, where the ophthalmic and angular veins cojoin (Fig. 2).

Secondary involvement of the third, fourth, fifth, and sixth cranial nerves may occur, with damage to them as they course through the cavernous sinus. Ophthalmoplegias are most frequently seen, with involvement of the abducens nerve (59%) (Fig. 4), oculomotor nerve (41%), or trochlear nerve (53%) (11). From review of

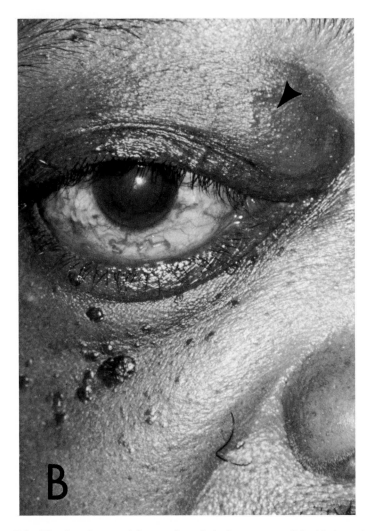

FIG. 2B. Prominence of the angular vein in the superomedial orbit *(arrow).*

the above percentages, it is evident that cranial ocular motor nerve pareses frequently occur in various combinations. Trigeminal involvement is also seen (29%). Other cranial nerves may be directly damaged by the initiating trauma. Involvement of the optic nerve (39%) and facial nerve (35%) occurs in this fashion.

Headache is reported to be of two types. An evanescent, throbbing, pulsatile pain (usually synchronous with the onset of the bruit) may occur, disappearing over several days to weeks. Others describe a chronic, constant, ipsilateral ocular and periorbital pain, with or without objective trigeminal hypalgesia (7,8).

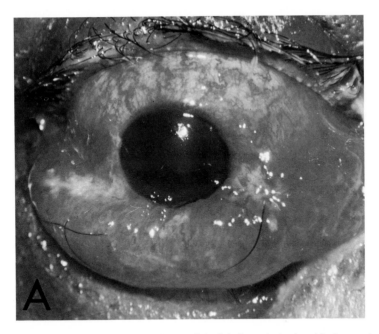

FIG. 3A. Advanced chemosis with prolapse of the inferior palpebral and bulbar conjunctiva.

Glaucoma has also been discovered to be of two distinct types. The aqueous humor in the anterior chamber of the eye is constantly being produced and must therefore be constantly drained. The trabecular meshwork in the angle of the anterior chamber drains aqueous humor through the canal of Schlemm, eventually reaching the episcleral venous network. Weekers and Demarcelle showed that the intraocular pressure rises in a millimeter for millimeter fashion, subsequent to the obligatory rise in episcleral venous pressure induced by a CCF (21). This type of glaucoma is seen in untreated, stable CCF, is often mild, and is frequently not difficult to control. The second type of glaucoma is far more serious. It is associated with a much higher intraocular pressure, a poor response to treatment, and with frequent visual loss. It is more often seen in chronic, poorly compensated cases of CCF, or in those treated with arterial occlusive or "trapping" procedures. Weiss noted the similarities of this form of glaucoma to the "neovascular" glaucoma seen in diabetes and in carotid or ophthalmic artery insufficiency (22). Under these conditions chronic hypoxia stimulates vigorous new vessel formation in many ocular tissues, including the region of the anterior chamber trabecular meshwork. The resultant obstruction of aqueous outflow produces a severe glaucoma which is difficult to control (15).

Miscellaneous ocular findings listed in Table 1 include corneal exposure keratopathy related to proptosis, incomplete lid closure, and associated fifth or seventh

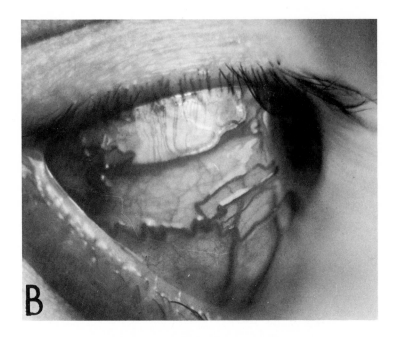

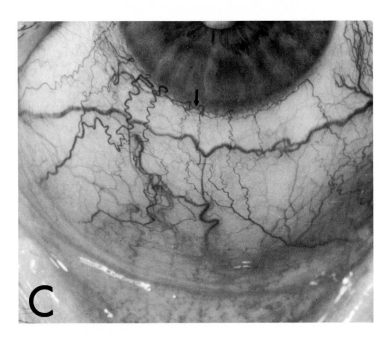

FIG. 3B and C. Prominent arterialized episcleral and conjunctival veins which are seen to extend to the limbus *(arrow).*

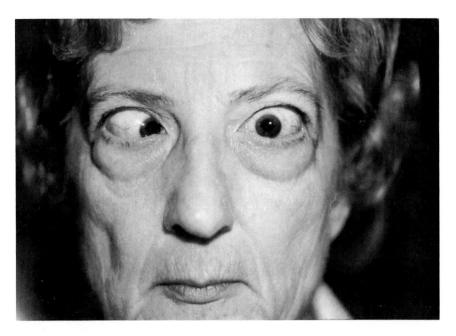

FIG. 4. Right abducens nerve palsy in carotid cavernous fistula.

cranial nerve involvement. The cornea may also appear generally cloudy or hazy. A focused beam of light shone through the anterior chamber may appear to be "passing through smoke," indicating a cell and flare reaction. The pupil may be dilated and fixed (or poorly reactive), and iris atrophy or synechiae connecting the posterior iris to the anterior lens surface may be seen. Lenticular opacities may occur. Venous engorgement and tortuosity are consistent ipsilateral retinal findings (Fig. 5). This may become more extreme and the picture of venous stasis retinopathy supervenes (Fig. 6). Venous distention, mild disk edema, and dot and blot hemorrhages appearing in the midzonal to peripheral retina, comprise the ophthalmoscopic picture. Retinal detachment rarely occurs. The optic nerve may exhibit disk edema, optic atrophy, glaucomatous cupping, or neovascularity. The central retinal artery frequently appears quite small and is rarely.occluded (15).

Visual loss is one of the most dreaded sequelae of CCF. The incidence of loss of vision in various reported series ranges from 50 to 89% (20). Visual loss may be an early or late finding. Early decline in vision is most often the result of corneal damage from exposure, or the result of direct traumatic damage to the globe or optic nerve. Late visual loss, however, is frequently secondary to absolute glaucoma or to corneal, lenticular, or retinal abnormalities described under "miscellaneous ocular findings" in Table 1. An understanding of the pathophysiology of late visual loss is critical in formulating effective therapeutic modalities that reduce visual morbidity. Knox (9) identified a syndrome of ocular findings encountered in chronic

TABLE 2. *Ocular findings in chronic hypoxia*

Cornea
Haze or edema
Anterior chamber
Cell and flare
Neovascularization of the angle
Glaucoma
Iris
Pupillary paralysis
Posterior synechiae
Iris atrophy
Lens
Cataract
Retina
Venous dilatation
Microaneurysms
Retinal hemorrhage
Optic disk
Optic atrophy
Ischemic optic neuropathy
Neovascularization
Glaucomatous cupping
Central retinal artery occlusion

eye to remain open, the intraluminal pressure must always remain higher than the intraocular pressure. Thus, the arteriovenous pressure gradient in the ocular circulation is normally the lowest in the carotid tree, and blood flow through the choroidal and central retinal arteries is correspondingly more fragile. Any other factors which arise that cause a further increase in ocular venous pressure, or a drop in ophthalmic artery pressure, will tend to decrease intraocular blood flow. If a critical arteriovenous pressure gradient is reached, ocular ischemia and hypoxia result. Such a set of complicating factors exists in the case of a CCF. The ophthalmic artery usually arises within or just above the cavernous sinus. With a fistulous opening from the carotid to the cavernous sinus, blood normally destined for the ophthalmic artery is diverted. In a very high-flow fistula, the flow may actually be reversed in the ophthalmic, as the CCF can "steal" blood from external carotid branches via external carotid–ophthalmic anastomoses. As the bulk of flow out of the cavernous sinus is usually directed anteriorly into the superior and inferior ophthalmic veins, the ocular venous system exists at a much higher pressure than normal. Thus the arterial pressure falls and the venous pressure rises, lowering the arteriovenous pressure gradient. The perfusion pressure of the ocular circulatory bed thus falls in an obligatory fashion, and ocular blood flow is rendered marginal or inadequate. If glaucoma develops, and especially if it is severe, further circulatory compromise occurs. The venous pressure of the eye must stay above the intraocular pressure in order to be patent, forcing a further millimeter for millimeter rise in venous pressure with increasing intraocular pressure. An eye suffering from borderline circulatory function may become profoundly hypoxic and ischemic as secondary glaucoma supervenes (15). In summary, with CCF, the ophthalmic artery blood flow is diverted into the fistula, thus lowering ophthalmic artery pressure. The ocular venous pressure is elevated, secondary to arterialization of the ocular veins that now drain the fistula, and to elevated intraocular pressure. The ocular arteriovenous pressure gradient drops and blood flow to the eye is rendered marginal or critically low. The high incidence of visual loss in CCF is, therefore, not surprising.

The aims of therapy for CCF are to obliterate the fistula, decreasing orbital congestive and circulatory symptoms produced by it, and at the same time to preserve vision. With older treatments, including carotid occlusive procedures and some "trapping" operations, the fistula often was incompletely obliterated secondary to the extensive collateralization of arterial supply. As might be predicted from the above discussion, visual loss was an unhappy and all too frequent complication of such procedures. With occlusion of the carotid artery from below, and at times above the cavernous sinus as well, the ophthalmic artery pressure may fall drastically. If the fistula is incompletely obliterated, the venous pressure may not fall as much as desired. The resultant ocular arteriovenous pressure gradient is lowered, and blood flow may be compromised below a critical level necessary to sustain the eye. Visual loss may unfortunately result. Newer techniques which preserve carotid artery flow (thus preserving ophthalmic artery pressure), while simultaneously decreasing the venous pressure in the superior ophthalmic vein, theoretically offer the best chance of reducing visual morbidity. Balloon embolization of the venous side of the fistula or electrothrombosis of the cavernous sinus are examples of techniques which theoretically protect the ocular arteriovenous circulatory gradient. Initial results using such techniques seem promising, but a careful documentation of neuro-ophthalmological outcome in patients so treated has yet to be published (1,5).

When treating patients with CCF, other general principles may be kept in mind, which may benefit ultimate visual outcome. Systemic measures may occasionally be quite helpful in assisting the ocular arteriovenous pressure gradient. Acceptance of moderate hypertension without vigorous treatment may indirectly help maintain ophthalmic artery pressure. Lowering blood viscosity when polycythemia, hyperlipidemia, or macroglobulinemia co-exist with CCF, may improve overall blood flow. Correction of an anemia, and vigorous treatment of lung disease, may improve tissue oxygenation significantly. During any hospital stay or operative procedure, blood pressure should be rigorously monitored, and hypotension promptly corrected. Correcting right-sided congestive heart failure may decrease venous pressure to some extent. Treatment of elevated intraocular pressure should be instituted early, with vigorous pursuit of correction of intraocular pressure to as normal a level as is safely possible. All of the above methods theoretically directly or indirectly improve ocular arteriovenous gradient and increase useful blood flow within the eye. These methods then give the surgeon maximum leeway in protecting the eye from the effects of ischemia, both before and after surgical or angiographic procedure to correct the fistula.

Spontaneous closure of traumatic CCF is rare. It was reported in 16 of the 322 cases reviewed by Sattler (16), and in only 4 of the 621 cases collected from the literature by Sugar and Meyer (17). Scattered reports of its occurrence have been more recently noted in the literature, with "spontaneous" closure most often following an angiographic procedure (13).

Spontaneous CCFs, although presenting in a similar clinical fashion as their traumatic counterparts, more frequently show incomplete or partial symptomatology. This fistula usually carries less blood, has a lower flow rate, and produces a milder elevation of pressure in the draining veins. Serious hypoxic/ischemic visual loss is less frequent. Although no firm figures are available, it is generally believed that these fistulas are more likely to recover spontaneously. In Newton and Hoyt's series of 11 patients with spontaneous carotid cavernous fistulae, only 1 suffered visual loss. Spontaneous closure occurred in 5 of the 11 patients, or 45% (12). Since the symptoms are frequently mild and incomplete, the incidence of visual loss lower, and the potential for spontaneous remission greater, many advocate cautious follow-up as the treatment of choice in such patients. Careful neurological and neuro-ophthalmological serial examinations with serial angiography may disclose improvement, and surgical or angiographic treatment can be avoided.

REFERENCES

1. Berenstein, A., Kricheff, I. I., and Ransohoff, J. (1980): Carotid cavernous fistulas: Intra-arterial treatment. *Am. J. Neuroradiol.*, 1:449–457.
2. Boyes, T. L., and Ralph, F. T. (1954): Carotid cavernous fistula. *Am. J. Ophthalmol.*, 37:262–266.
3. Brismar, G., and Brismar, J. (1976): Spontaneous carotid cavernous fistulas. *Acta Ophthalmol.*, 54:542–552.
4. Bynke, H. G., and Efsing, H. O. (1970): Carotid cavernous fistula with contralateral exophthalmos. *Acta Ophthalmol.*, 48:971–978.
5. Debrun, G., Lacour, P., Caron, J. P., and Keravel, Y. (1978): Detachable balloon and calibrated-leak balloon techniques in the treatment of cerebral vascular lesions. *J. Neurosurg.*, 49:635–649.
6. Graf, C. J. (1965): Spontaneous carotid cavernous fistula: Ehlers-Danlos syndrome and related conditions. *Arch. Neurol.*, 13:664–672.
7. Hamby, W. B., and Dohn, D. D. (1965): Carotid cavernous fistulas: Report of thirty-six cases. *Clin. Neurosurg.*, 11:150–170.
8. Henderson, J. W., and Schneider, R. C. (1959): The ocular findings in carotid cavernous fistula. *Am. J. Ophthalmol.*, 48:585–597.
9. Knox, D. L. (1969): Ocular aspects of cervical vascular disease. *Surv. Ophthalmol.*, 13:245–260.
10. Locke, C. E., Jr. (1924): Arteriovenous aneurysm or pulsating exophthalmos. *Ann. Surg.*, 80:1–33.
11. Martin, J. D., and Mabon, R. F. (1943): Pulsating exophthalmos. *J.A.M.A.*, 121:330–334.
12. Newton, T. H., and Hoyt, W. F. (1970): Arteriovenous shunts in the region of the cavernous sinus. *Neuroradiology*, 1:71–81.
13. Potter, J. M. (1954): Carotid cavernous fistula: Five cases with "spontaneous" recovery. *Br. Med. J.*, 2:786–788.
14. Rios-Montenegro, E. N., Behrens, M. M., and Hoyt, W. F. (1972): Pseudoxanthoma elasticum, association with unilateral carotid cavernous fistula. *J. Neurosurg.*, 25:151–155.
15. Sanders, M. D., and Hoyt, W. F. (1969): Hypoxic ocular sequelae of carotid cavernous fistulae. *Br. J. Ophthalmol.*, 53:82–97.
16. Sattler, C. H. (1920): In: *Handbuch der Gesamten Augenheilkunde*, edited by A. Graefe and T. Saemisch, Vol. 9, chapter 13. W. Engelmann, Leipzig.
17. Sugar, H. S., and Meyer, S. J. (1940): Pulsating exophthalmos. *Arch. Ophthalmol.*, 23:1288–1321.
18. Takahashi, M., Killeffer, F., and Wilson, G. (1969): Iatrogenic carotid cavernous fistula. *J. Neurosurg.*, 30:498–502.
19. Walker, A. E., and Allegre, G. E. (1956): Carotid cavernous fistulas. *Surgery*, 39:411–422.

20. Walsh, F. B., and Hoyt, W. F. editors (1968): *Clinical Neuro-ophthalmology*, pp. 1714–1737. The Williams and Wilkins Co., Baltimore.
21. Weekers, R., and Delmarcelle, Y. (1952): Pathogenesis of intraocular tension in cases of arteriovenous aneurysm. *Arch. Ophthalmol.*, 48:338–343.
22. Weiss, D. L., Shaffer, R. M., and Nehrenberg, T. R. (1963): Neovascular glaucoma complicating carotid cavernous fistula. *Arch. Ophthalmol.*, 69:304–307.

Vascular Malformations, edited by
R.R. Smith, A. Haerer and W.F. Russell.
Raven Press, New York © 1982.

Treatment of Carotid Cavernous and Vertebral Fistulas

Gerard Debrun

Section of Neuroradiology, University Hospital, London, Ontario N6A 5A5

CAROTID CAVERNOUS FISTULAS

The first reported case of carotid cavernous fistula was a cavernous aneurysm that had ruptured into the cavernous sinus, published by Benjamin Travers in 1811. However, it was thought that the cause of the pulsating exophthalmos in this patient was an aneurysm of the cavernous carotid siphon.

Baron of France presented before the Anatomical Society of Paris in 1935 the first specimen of an aneurysm of the internal carotid artery ruptured into the cavernous sinus.

Delens, in his thesis of 1970, reported two of Nelaton's cases of traumatic carotid cavernous fistulas.

The earlier cases were treated by carotid ligation, but the mortality was very high and few were cured.

ETIOLOGY

Carotid cavernous fistulas may be spontaneous or traumatic. Spontaneous cases are more prevalent in women and elderly people. Pregnancy seems to have some influence on their onset. Traumatic cases occur with equal frequency in men and women; this was not true some decades ago when men were more exposed to trauma than women. Traumatic fistulas are, in fact, a rare complication of all significant head injuries. They are often associated with basal skull fractures and, rarely, with a penetrating injury through the orbit.

In spontaneous cases, some fistulas probably develop from rupture of a preexisting subclinoid aneurysm. However, although a cavernous aneurysm is not unusual, a complicating fistula is exceptional.

Sugar proposed that the remnant of the primitive trigeminal artery might cause an aneurysm at this site. In fact, no documented case of fistula associated with a trigeminal artery has been published.[1] Most spontaneous cases are more likely a type of dural arteriovenous malformation (AVM) in view of the rich anastomotic

---

[1]Since the writing of this chapter, we have become aware of two cases of carotid cavernous fistula associated with a trigeminal artery.

plexus that normally exists between meningeal branches of the carotid siphon and the external carotid artery.

In such cases, selective angiography of the internal carotid artery demonstrates many tiny branches from the carotid siphon opacifying the cavernous sinus. It is impossible to enter the cavernous sinus with a balloon, which is not indicated for treatment of this type of fistula. Similarly, many meningeal branches from the internal maxillary artery and its meningeal branches, and occasionally from the ascending pharyngeal artery, can be shown on hyperselective angiography of external carotid branches. The treatment of spontaneous fistulas consists of embolization of these branches with particles or bucrylate.

Bilateral carotid cavernous fistulas are not rare, with cross-filling from one side to the other, there being no logical correlation with the side of the exophthalmos.

In traumatic cases, arterial rents of 2 to 4 mm have been demonstrated. In the first case of Nelaton in Delen's thesis, the artery was almost completely divided by the splinter of bone.

Anatomical specimens are rare and difficult to study. In 1950, Taptas reviewed 48 autopsy cases. He could not find the communication in 22 of these cases and concluded erroneously that a communication did not exist in all cases.

In most cases the hole of the fistula is on the posterior ascending portion of the cavernous carotid or on the horizontal portion.

The fact that the opening of the fistula can be occluded with a single balloon proves that the opening is unique (Fig. 1, B and C). However, in my experience of 52 cases of traumatic carotid cavernous fistulas, there were 2 cases where the cavernous sinus could be entered through two different openings. Traumatic fistulas with many torn branches of the siphon are probably very uncommon. As these branches are normally anastomosed to meningeal branches of the external carotid artery, selective external angiography is necessary even in traumatic cases. It will be normal in most cases. The venous drainage depends partially on the location of the fistula. Anterior fistulas cause the most impressive exophthalmos, and the ophthalmic veins are widely distended (Fig. 1A). When the fistula is posterior, the exophthalmos can be minimal even with a huge shunt. The superior and inferior petrosal sinuses are widely open. Frequently, the contralateral cavernous sinus fills (Fig. 2B).

From the size of the cavernous sinus seen on the angiogram, it is impossible to predict the size of the fistula and the number of balloons that will be needed to occlude it because partitions within the sinus may be overlooked. Casts of the normal cavernous sinus have shown a plexus of veins, but in a case of carotid cavernous fistula these veins are extremely dilated, and the partitions of the sinus more or less ruptured, especially in long-standing untreated cases. The angiogram only shows the overall size of the cavernous sinus when the shunt is rapid. It is only at the time of treatment with a balloon catheter that one learns how many balloons are needed to occlude the fistula. Similarly unknown in advance is the volume of the balloon necessary, even if only one is needed to occlude the fistula.

CLINICAL PRESENTATION BEFORE TREATMENT

Traumatic Cavernous Fistula

Pulsating exophthalmos and bruit appear immediately or weeks after trauma. Exophthalmos, edema of the eyelids, and chemosis are sometimes very impressive and more severe than in spontaneous cases. Pictures of the eye must be taken before treatment. Diplopia is often present due to paresis of the sixth nerve. Less often there is complete ophthalmoplegia with paresis of the fourth and third nerves. These findings must be carefully noted before treatment which may itself induce oculomotor palsy. Some patients complain of pain in the orbital and sinus areas from irritation of the fifth nerve. This subjective feeling must also be noted initially because treatment may induce retro-orbital and facial pain during the ensuing weeks. Vision remains normal for weeks or months and then gradually decreases. It is important to note the degree of vision at the time of treatment. Rarely, the optic nerve will have been damaged by a spur of bone, and the eye will be blind.

Spontaneous Carotid Cavernous Fistula

Pulsating exophthalmos, chemosis, and bruit are often minimal. Bilateral fistulas are encountered more often than in traumatic cases. In this type of fistula, there is often contralateral venous drainage and pulsating exophthalmos on that side; this does not prove that the fistula is on that side. Internal and external selective angiograms on both sides are absolutely necessary. When treatment has to be decided because of intolerable pain, bruit, progressive loss of vision, or oculomotor nerve palsy, one must always keep in mind that spontaneous healing occurs more frequently with spontaneous than with traumatic fistulas.

RADIOLOGICAL EVALUATION

As vertebral angiography is always necessary, the radiological evaluation of a carotid cavernous fistula (Figs. 1A, 1B, and 2) is best achieved by Seldinger's technique through the femoral artery. A heparin-coated 5F catheter is directed to the internal carotid artery on the side of the pulsating exophthalmos and bruit. Ten milliliters of contrast material is injected in 1 sec with an automatic syringe. Lateral films can be coned on the area of interest. Anteroposterior films are coned transorbital veins. The number of films per second depends on many factors. In the institutions where magnification is routinely used, no more than two films per second might be taken. With most film changers, without magnification, it is risky to get more than four films per second, exceptionally six films per second. With this cadence, the cavernous sinus fills very quickly and the exact location of the fistula can hardly be determined. It is possible to analyze the type of venous drainage anteriorly, with big ophthalmic veins, and posteriorly, with big inferior and superior petrosal veins or both. It is also worthwhile to note that some fistulas with a rapid, massive steal

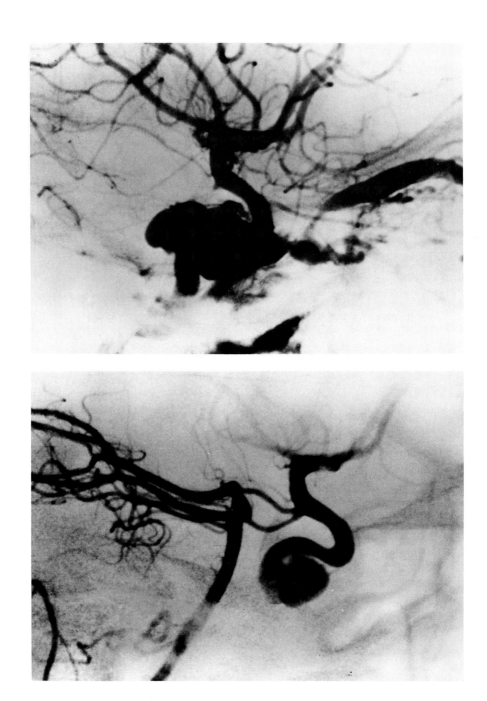

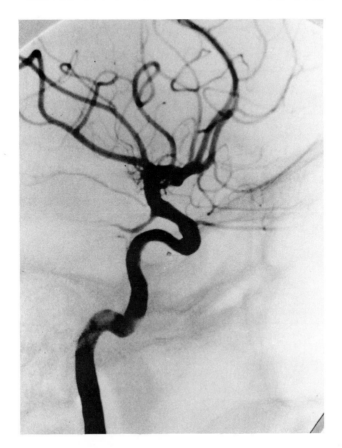

FIG. 1 (A to C). Traumatic carotid cavernous fistula. One hole. One balloon. **A** (top). Right internal carotid artery. Big cavernous sinus. **B** (bottom). Vertebral angiography with compression of the right carotid in the neck. Retrograde opacification of the siphon, then of the fistula and of the cavernous sinus. **C.** One balloon has been detached in the cavernous sinus. The balloon is inflated with silicone. It totally occludes the hole. The carotid artery is well preserved. Same stable result 6 months later.

fail to opacify the internal carotid artery above the level of the fistula (Fig. 2A). In such a case the location of the fistula is easier to predict, but it would be a mistake to think that the internal carotid is not functional above the level of the fistula, and that the only treatment would be to occlude the siphon at the level of the fistula with a Fogarty catheter without trying to save the carotid artery. It would be risky to embolize the fistula through the internal carotid artery without clipping the carotid artery at the level of the ophthalmic artery. One can recognize this risk by getting a vertebral angiogram or contralateral carotid angiogram with compression of the carotid artery on the side of the fistula (Fig. 2, C and D). In most cases, the fistula gets blood from above through the posterior communicating artery, the anterior communicating artery, or both, and the carotid siphon above the level of the fistula is retrogradely opacified to the level of the fistula, as illustrated in Fig. 2D.

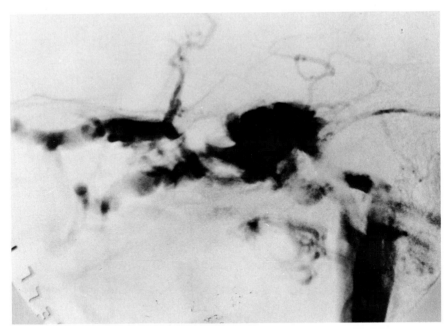

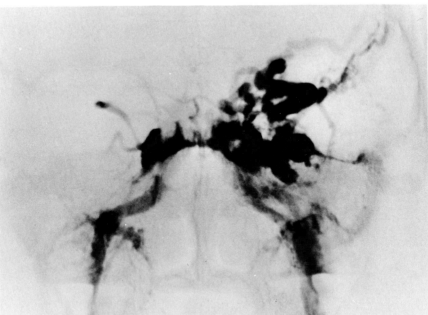

FIG. 2A (top) and **B** (bottom).   Left traumatic carotid cavernous fistula. Total steal. The internal carotid artery above the fistula is not opacified. This does not prove that it is occluded. Venous drainage is through superior and inferior orbital veins, inferior petrosal sinus, pterygoid plexus, sylvian vein, and contralateral cavernous sinus.

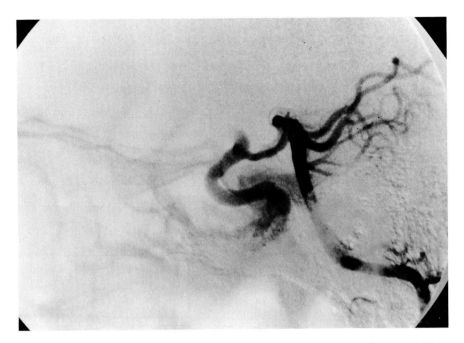

FIG. 2C. Left vertebral angiogram with compression of the left carotid artery in the neck. Now, the internal carotid artery fills retrogradely and demonstrates the level of the fistula.

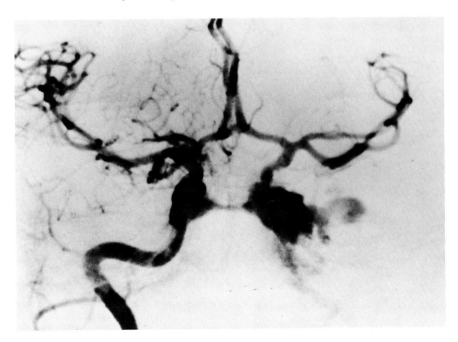

FIG. 2D. Contralateral carotid angiogram with compression of the carotid artery.

A contralateral carotid angiogram and vertebral angiogram with homolateral compression of the carotid artery are needed to demonstrate the location and size of the fistula and to demonstrate the quality of the communicating arteries if one wishes to occlude the carotid siphon (Fig. 2, C and D). The aim of modern treatment of a fistula is always to save the carotid artery, either by a detachable-balloon technique or by operation on the cavernous sinus.

It is possible to demonstrate the size and the place of the fistula at the time of treatment. When a wide introducer (7F or 8F) is in the internal carotid artery, one can use a double-lumen 5F balloon catheter which is maneuvered inside the introducer. The balloon is inflated above the tip of the introducer at the C2 or C3 level until it occludes the internal carotid (Fig. 3B). Contrast material is injected through the other lumen and slowly fills the fistula. This technique is indicated

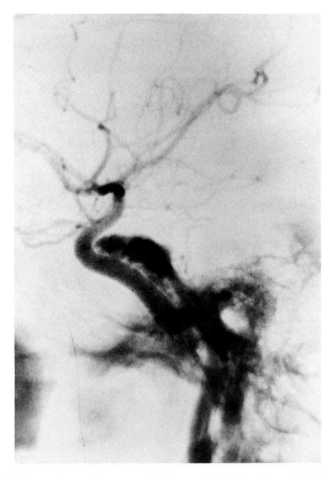

FIG. 3A.   Left traumatic carotid cavernous fistula, venous drainage through the inferior petrosal sinus.

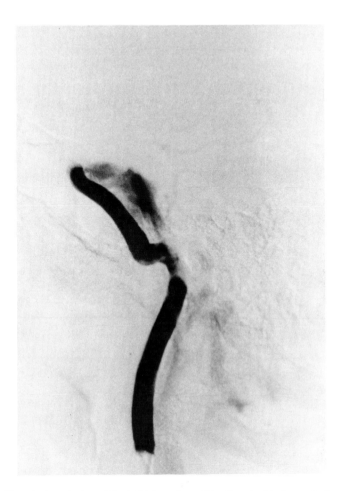

FIG. 3B. Transient occlusion of the left internal carotid with a double-lumen balloon catheter. The hole of the fistula is small and difficult to penetrate with a balloon introduced into the artery.

when the posterior or anterior communicating artery does not exist. During attempts to enter the fistula with the balloon, if the cavernous sinus is not immediately penetrated with the detachable balloon, one can inflate it at different levels of the carotid siphon and every time inject some contrast material into the carotid artery. If the balloon is inflated below the fistula or occludes it, the angiogram will show occlusion of the internal carotid artery. If the balloon is above the fistula, the angiogram will show that the flow is preserved with rapid opacification of the cavernous sinus. Bilateral external carotid angiograms are also necessary. In traumatic cases the external carotid angiogram is generally normal. In the rare cases where small siphon branches are torn in the cavernous sinus, the distal branches of the carotid can be demonstrated. With spontaneous fistulas some tiny branches of the carotid siphon communicate with the cavernous sinus and are demonstrated

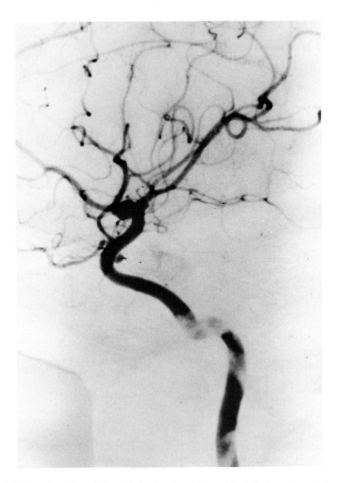

FIG. 3C.   A balloon introduced through the jugular vein and the inferior petrosal sinus has been detached in the cavernous sinus. The fistula is occluded with a minimal leak at the level of the fistula, mimicking a false aneurysm.

by selective internal carotid angiogram. There are also often tiny meningeal vessels from the internal maxillary artery demonstrated by hyperselective external angiograms. Injection of hypertonic contrast material in the external carotid artery is painful; isotonic contrast material is tolerated more comfortably. An injection speed of 4 to 6 ml per sec is sufficiently rapid, with a total injection of 8 ml. The degree of participation of carotid siphon and external carotid branches varies from case to case. In some instances, the only feeders of the fistula are branches of the external carotid artery, possibly including the occipital or the ascending pharyngeal artery, less often the middle meningeal artery and distal branches of the internal maxillary artery.

As a last point in the evaluation of a carotid cavernous fistula, the status of the bifurcation of the carotid artery must be carefully noted, because stenosis or distorted origin of the internal carotid would complicate the catheterization. In the same way, severe kinking or a complete loop of the internal carotid artery in the neck are of major importance, because treatment with a balloon catheter then becomes much more difficult and risky. On rare occasions, the internal carotid in the neck has been dissected by an injury, and this lesion could be a contraindication to balloon catheterization.

TREATMENT OF TRAUMATIC CAROTID CAVERNOUS FISTULA

Many different types of procedures have been proposed and can be divided into two groups. The first group consists of procedures to occlude the fistula with sacrifice of the internal carotid artery. One type is ligation of the internal carotid artery at the level of the anterior clinoid process, with or without ligation of the ophthalmic artery, but with embolization of the fistula through the internal carotid artery. Another procedure is occlusion of the carotid siphon with a nondetachable balloon (Fogarty or Prolo's catheter) or with a detachable balloon. The balloon is long enough to occlude the neck of the fistula and the cavernous portion of the carotid artery completely. These procedures are possible when the anterior or posterior communicating arteries are wide open. Otherwise, if the patient does not tolerate occlusion of the carotid artery, an external-internal by-pass has to be performed before occlusion of the siphon.

The second group of procedures occlude the fistula and save the carotid artery. These techniques have been made possible by improvements in the surgical approach to the cavernous sinus, in anesthesiology, and in hyperselective catheterization of external and internal carotid arteries.

In regard to the surgical approach to the cavernous sinus, Mullan (7) has demonstrated that the cavernous sinus could be packed by different techniques, through the superior ophthalmic vein at its entrance to the cavernous sinus when the fistula is anterior, or through the superior petrosal sinus when the fistula drains posteriorly (Fig. 3A). The lateral wall of the cavernous sinus can be punctured with small needles and the sinus packed with phosphor-bronze wire. The neck of the fistula can be occluded with thrombogenic needles. These techniques induce thrombosis of the cavernous sinus with occlusion of the fistula. They are simpler than direct ligation of the fistula done in some cases by Parkinson (8) but with deep hypothermia and under cardiac arrest. Charles Drake has also successfully treated cavernous fistulas by packing the cavernous sinus with pieces of muscle.

As to intravascular navigation with a balloon catheter, the cavernous sinus can be reached with a balloon catheter maneuvered through the veins or through the internal carotid artery.

When the superior ophthalmic vein is widely dilated, it could be desirable to reach the cavernous sinus by percutaneous puncture or cut-down of the angular vein. I have always failed to pass all the curves of the superior ophthalmic vein with a balloon catheter. However, Peterson et al. (9) treated some patients with catheterization of the superior ophthalmic vein with an insulated copper wire. When the inferior petrosal sinus is dilated in a case of posterior fistula, it is possible to catheterize the origin of the petrosal vein with the balloon catheter bent at the tip. The jugular vein has to be catheterized either from the femoral vein with a 90-cm introducer or through the neck by direct puncture of the jugular vein and catheterization with a sheath (type Cordis) number 7 or 8F. The introducer is then easily maneuvered through the sheath. When the inferior petrosal sinus has been reached, it becomes easy to proceed retrogradely to the cavernous sinus with the balloon catheter. Mullan (7) successfully treated one patient by this method with occlusion of the fistula and preservation of the internal carotid. Some authors have reported occlusions of the fistula with a Fogarty catheter introduced through the jugular vein. I have closed one fistula with a balloon detached in the cavernous sinus through the inferior petrosal sinus (Fig. 3C). It is often easy to get to the cavernous sinus but difficult to push the balloon close to the fistula because of the partitions or narrow portions of the cavernous sinus.

When the venous drainage of the fistula is predominantly posterior with a dilated inferior petrosal sinus of 3 mm diameter or more, the first step of the treatment should be an attempt to occlude the fistula from the venous side, an extremely elegant and safe procedure.

BALLOON CATHETER MANEUVER THROUGH THE INTERNAL CAROTID ARTERY

Two different types of balloon catheters can be used with two totally different techniques. One is the detachable balloon catheter first described by Serbinenko (10), then modified and used by myself (1,2). The second is a Silastic balloon catheter which cannot be detached but which has a calibrated leak at the tip and permits the delivery of a polymerizing acrylic substance, bucrylate (isobutyl-2-cyanoacrylate), solidifying instantaneously when it is in contact with blood.

THE DETACHABLE-BALLOON TECHNIQUE

The balloons are made from latex sleeves of different sizes (Fig. 4). The diameter of the sleeve varies from 0.3 to 2 mm. The length of the sleeve is also variable, with long or short cylindrical balloons or even round balloons. Some sleeves have an additional flap at the tip when a small silver cylinder of 0.7 or 1 mm in diameter can be lodged. The balloon can be followed on the fluoroscopic screen without having to be inflated with iodine contrast material. Most of the sleeves have a narrow proximal portion that grips the catheter and the balloon itself will be made of the distal expansible portion.

There are two basic types of detachable balloon. Type I (Fig. 5) in which the balloon is only held on the catheter by a narrow portion of the sleeve, requires no second coaxial catheter for detachment, but is not self-sealing and can only be used with a polymerizing substance. Type II, in which the balloon is tied to the catheter with latex thread, requires a second coaxial catheter for detachment but is self-sealing and can be used with iodine contrast material or polymerizing substance as well (Fig. 6).

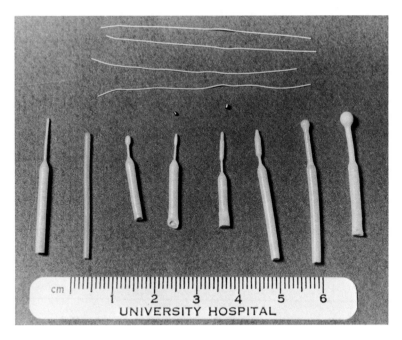

FIG. 4. Different types of latex sleeves. Four latex threads. Two silver cylinders which can be lodged in the narrow distal tip of sleeves numbers 4, 5, and 6.

TYPE I BALLOON CATHETER

The narrow portion of the sleeve simply grips the catheter through its own elasticity. One can invaginate the narrow portion into the balloon so that it grips the catheter more tightly.

The advantages of this type of balloon are:

a) The balloon is detached by simply pulling on the catheter.

b) A thin-walled, elastic, and supple polyethylene catheter can be used because the balloon is not strongly tied to the catheter (0.25 mm internal 0.50 mm external diameter).

The disadvantages of this balloon type are:

a) There is a real danger of detaching the balloon prematurely by, for example, pulling the catheter inadvertently.

b) This balloon cannot be detached when filled with iodine contrast material because it would leak and deflate immediately. When the capacity of the balloon needed to occlude the fistula has been measured with iodine contrast material, this quantity must be removed and replaced with an equal quantity of polymerizing substance. When this substance has solidified, detachment is performed by pulling the catheter. At that time there are three dangers. The first is that the balloon does

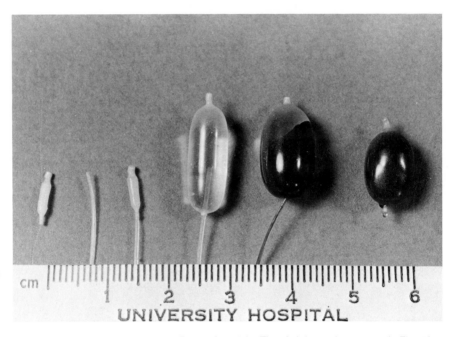

FIG. 5.   Detachable balloon type I. From left to right: The sixth latex sleeve seen in Fig. 4 has been cut, keeping 2 mm of the narrow portion. The silver cylinder has been placed in the tip. Teflon tubing 0.4 × 0.6 mm or polyethylene tubing 0.25 × 0.50 mm. After dilatation of the narrow portion with a forceps, the tubing has entered the sleeve. The balloon can be inflated with iodine contrast. After deflating the balloon and measuring its capacity, an equal quantity of silicone mixed with tantalum powder is injected. The quantity of iodine contrast material which was inside the catheter and could not be aspirated (dead space), has been reintroduced into the balloon. When silicone has solidified, the Teflon catheter is pulled out, the balloon is detached and generally loses its iodine contrast component.

not stay in the cavernous sinus and moves into the carotid artery through the neck of the fistula. The second is damage to the neck of the fistula. The third is that a small bulge of solidified silicone forms at the neck of the balloon. The first danger is by far the greatest.

c) This type of non-self-sealing balloon cannot be used when a balloon inflated with iodine contrast material must be detached. This occurs in three conditions explained below.

TYPE II BALLOON CATHETER

The balloon is firmly tied to the catheter with an elastic latex thread. Polyethylene tubing is not strong enough and would lengthen or rupture at the time of detachment of the balloon when the catheter is pulled. Instead, thin-walled Teflon tubing (0.4 mm internal and 0.6 mm external diameter) is used. The catheter to which the balloon is tied is called catheter A. It becomes slightly smaller and more supple by lengthening it from 130 to 150 cm. In order to detach the balloon (which, with

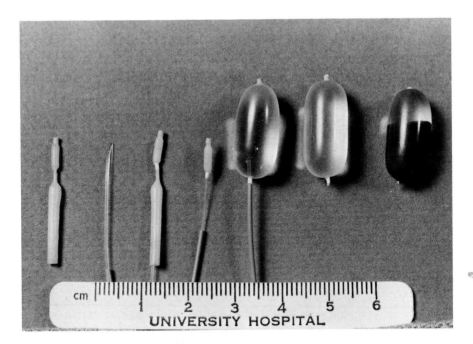

FIG. 6. Detachable balloon type II. From left to right: Sleeve with silver cylinder in its tip. Teflon tubing 0.4 × 0.6 mm. The coaxial polyethylene tubing is seen at the lower part of the Teflon tubing. The sleeve has been ligated over the Teflon tubing with a latex thread. The lower part of the sleeve below the ligature has been cut. The polyethylene coaxial catheter is visible. The balloon is inflated with iodine contrast material (Conray 60 or Hypaque 60). The polyethylene coaxial catheter now reaches the ligature and allows pulling out of the Teflon tubing without dislodging the balloon. After detachment, the elasticity of the ligature closes the aperture of the balloon which does not leak. If silicone has been used, the balloon is partially filled with iodine and partially with silicone.

this type, could not be detached by simply pulling on the catheter), a second coaxial polyethylene catheter (called B) is slid up over catheter A until it is in contact with the base of the balloon, that is, the base of the ligature. Catheter B holds the balloon in place when catheter A is withdrawn to detach it.

The advantages of this balloon type are:

a. There is minimal risk of detaching the balloon prematurely because it is solidly tied to the catheter.

b. The balloon is self-sealing, because the elasticity of the thread is such that it closes the hole of the balloon when catheter A is withdrawn. This balloon can be filled with iodine contrast material and detached as soon as the proper capacity of the balloon is reached. There are three situations where such a balloon is needed. First, when the capacity of the balloon needed to occlude the fistula is less than or equal to the dead space of the single-lumen catheter A (Fig. 7). Second, when the balloon is difficult to lodge at the proper place to occlude the fistula and is drawn away by the flow when it is deflated. It becomes risky to inject a polymerizing substance which could solidify before the balloon has been correctly located. Third, when many balloons are needed to close the fistula. If all the balloons are filled with a polymerizing substance, the cavernous sinus may remain under pressure. Oculomotor palsies may occur, as may severe pain. The final result is much better if all the balloons except the last one are filled with iodine contrast material, because they will progressively return to normal size. The oculomotor palsies, if any, will improve more quickly.

The major disadvantage of this type of balloon is the need of a second coaxial catheter B to detach the balloon.

SINGLE-LUMEN CATHETER A OR DOUBLE-LUMEN CATHETER A

The problem of the dead space of the catheter has already been exposed (Fig. 7). With a single-lumen catheter, it would be best to start with injection of a low-viscous radiopaque polymerizing substance that would remain liquid until some drops of catalyst could be added. This, however, is impractical because the proportion of polymerizing substance and catalyst must be very precise and well mixed.

A double-lumen catheter (Fig. 8) allows one to work with iodine material as long as necessary, and then to inject the polymerizing substance through one lumen while the iodine contrast material previously in this lumen is pushed into the balloon and immediately aspirated through the second lumen. Manipulation is very precise and delicate, but the final result is a balloon totally filled with the solidified polymerizing substance, whatever its size.

The disadvantage of a double-lumen catheter will always be its size and its rigidity compared to a single-lumen catheter.

Because of the external diameter of the double-lumen catheter, close to 1 mm, a coaxial catheter is difficult to use. The latex sleeve is cut transversely at the level of the narrow portion of which 2-mm are kept. The narrow portion is dilated with a forceps, and the double-lumen catheter is introduced into the balloon. The 2-mm narrow portion grips the catheter. It is a type I balloon catheter with all its advantages and disadvantages.

BALLOONS FILLED WITH IODINE MATERIAL OR WITH POLYMERIZING SUBSTANCE

A latex balloon filled with iodine material and detached progressively deflates over a variable period of time, probably depending on the strength of the ligature. Most balloons are completely deflated 6 weeks after detachment. Experimental work has shown that a latex balloon filled with iodine material, isoosmolar with plasma, does not leak if it has been tied to the catheter with a long and solid ligature sufficiently strong so that the balloon could not be detached with the coaxial catheter without rupturing the Teflon catheter A.

The fistula is always occluded because of thrombosis of the cavernous sinus around the balloon, but in 50% of cases a false aneurysm or venous pouch appears in place of the deflated balloon (Fig. 9). Three complications may occur:

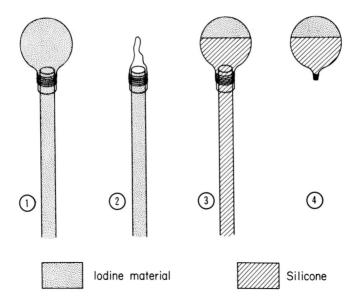

| Iodine material | | Silicone |

FIG. 7. Dead space of a single-lumen balloon catheter **1.** Balloon inflated with iodine contrast material; **2.** Balloon deflated. The iodine contrast material inside the catheter cannot be aspirated. It is the dead space of the catheter. **3.** When a polymerizing substance is injected, the iodine contrast material in the dead space of the catheter is pushed into the balloon again. If the capacity of the balloon needed to treat the lesion is equal to the capacity of the dead space, a polymerizing substance cannot be used. The balloon has to be of Type II, inflated with iodine contrast material and not leaking after detachment because of the elastic thread ligature.

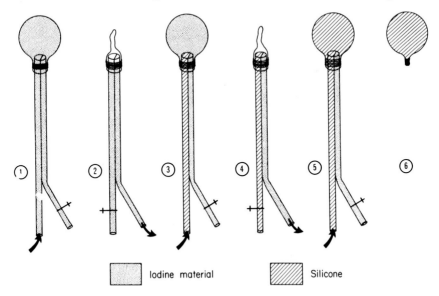

| Iodine material | | Silicone |

FIG. 8. Double-lumen catheter permits detaching a balloon only filled with polymerizing substance. **1.** Both lumens, as well as the balloon, contain iodine contrast material. **2.** The balloon is deflated through the left lumen, the capacity of which is known. **3.** Same volume of polymerizing substance is injected through the left lumen. The iodine contrast material contained in this lumen again enters the balloon but can be aspirated through the right lumen (as in **4**). **4.** When the balloon is empty of iodine material, injection of polymerizing substance starts again through the left lumen until (**5**) the balloon contains the appropriate volume.

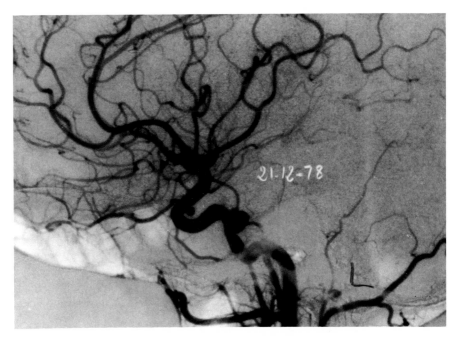

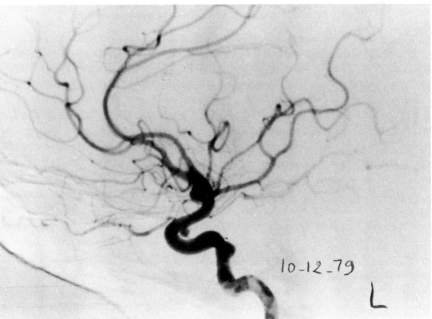

FIG. 10. A (top).   Left traumatic carotid cavernous sinus fistula 1 month after occlusion with an iodine inflated balloon. False aneurysm. **B** (bottom). Same patient. One year later, the false aneurysm is smaller. Asymptomatic patient. Incidental small cavernous aneurysm.

THE INTRODUCER

Whatever balloon catheter is used (single-lumen catheter A with its coaxial catheter B, or double-lumen catheter A alone), an additional catheter will be introduced into the internal carotid artery. The internal diameter catheter C has to be wide enough to allow easy maneuvers of catheters A and B as well as continuous infusion of heparinized saline and intermittent injections of iodine material (Fig. 11). Its size depends on the size of the biggest balloon needed. An inner diameter of 1.7 to 2 mm is usually sufficient. A thin-walled polyethylene catheter can be used with a wall of 0.2 mm. This introducer C easily passes through an 8F Cordis sheath placed in the femoral artery. The introducer is 90 cm long and is straight so that its tip is exactly in the center of the lumen of the internal carotid artery. A bent tip would adhere to the wall of the artery with the risk of clot formation and difficult maneuvers of the balloon catheter. The straight introducer C will enter the common carotid artery with one of the following three techniques:

a) With a 0.52-inch C guide; b) with a guide and bent-tip polyethylene catheter exactly fitting within the introducer; and c) with a 250-cm guide first placed in the carotid artery and along which the introducer will slide.

The introducer is connected to a side arm (Fig. 11). The balloon catheter enters the straight path of the side arm where a valve prevents bleeding along the catheter. A three-way stopcock is connected to the lateral path of the side arm, giving two additional paths, one for continuous heparinized infusion, the other for iodine contrast injections.

If for some reason (atherosclerosis of the femoral or iliac arteries on both sides, tortuous and dilated aortic arch) it is impossible to catheterize the common carotid from the femoral artery, the common carotid artery is punctured in the neck with an 18-gauge needle. An 8F sheath 20 cm long with a guide and a dilator is introduced into the common carotid artery and then directed to the internal carotid artery. This technique is difficult and dangerous with risk of damage to the wall of the internal carotid artery with the guide, especially if there is a loop in the cervical portion of the internal carotid. It is safer to direct the guide to the external carotid artery to avoid dissection of the internal carotid artery. The internal carotid artery, if damaged by the guide, goes into spasm and the procedure can fail and cause thrombosis of the internal carotid artery. The advantage of this technique is the decrease of the dead space of the catheter, which can be much shorter.

LOCAL ANESTHESIA OR GENERAL ANESTHESIA

All procedures can be done through the groin under local anesthesia. If the patient is very anxious, neuroleptanalgesia with the permanent presence of an anesthetist will be necessary. The patient will be quiet and relaxed but will be able to follow simple requests.

If the approach is through the neck, anesthesia with tracheal intubation is necessary, especially if systemic heparinization is used, because of the risk of sudden cervical hematoma formation after removal of the introducer.

of the balloon faces the presumed entrance of the fistula. The silver tip at this time is generally moved by a quick alternating motion. Some inflation and deflation of the balloon can help the balloon to enter the fistula. When these maneuvers fail, it is dangerous to persist and advisable to use a smaller balloon. If this balloon also fails to enter the fistula, the smallest balloon is used. Inability to enter the cavernous sinus is unusual.

When the piece of silver is believed to be in the cavernous sinus, the balloon is progressively inflated with iodine contrast material. From time to time an injection of iodine contrast material in the internal carotid artery demonstrates whether the fistula is totally occluded. The balloon is never filled to greater than its maximum known capacity. If its shape becomes biloculated, a partition in the cavernous sinus is squeezing the balloon with a risk of rupture. If the biggest balloon entering the cavernous sinus does not occlude the neck of the fistula even at maximum inflation, the cavernous pouch is large and needs more than one balloon. The first balloon is filled with iodine and detached. Then a second balloon of the same size is used immediately. If it does not occlude the fistula, it is detached and a third balloon is used, and so on, until the neck of the fistula is occluded without any leak of contrast material into the cavernous sinus. The last balloon is filled with silicone if possible; that is, a double-lumen balloon catheter is used at the end of the treatment or the balloon is partially filled with silicone with a single-lumen catheter. This depends on the ease with which the cavernous sinus is entered, and whether it is reasonable to exchange the last single-lumen balloon catheter for a double-lumen balloon catheter. If the last balloon can be totally filled with silicone, no venous pseudo-aneurysm will occur. If the balloon has been totally filled with iodine or partially filled with silicone, a pseudoaneurysm will occur in 50% of cases. With experience, one can avoid doing an angiogram prior to balloon detachment and look for sub-tracted films when the balloon occludes the neck of the fistula. This saves time.

DETACHMENT OF THE BALLOON

With a tied balloon, the coaxial catheter B is needed to detach the balloon safely. Catheter B is pushed up so that it slides along catheter A until it reaches the base of the balloon. It can be very difficult in some cases to slide the B catheter, especially when there is a loop of 180° of the internal carotid artery in the neck. To be sure that the coaxial catheter has reached the base of the balloon, the 30 cm of difference of length which exists between the coaxial B catheter (120 cm) and the Teflon A catheter (150 cm) must be found before trying to detach the balloon. Sometimes, when the sphenoidal sinus is widely aerated, the end of the coaxial B catheter is well seen on the screen. Subtraction television helps to visualize it. The coaxial B catheter is then held with the left hand and the Teflon catheter A is pulled out gently until the balloon is detached. This is done under fluoroscopy. The balloon does not move and does not deflate if the ligature works correctly. Detachment is successful if the operator can feel precisely when he detaches the balloon, but nothing is visible on the screen.

With an untied balloon and a double-lumen catheter, several manipulations are necessary before detachment. A 1-ml syringe is filled with catalyzed silicone (the mixture starts to solidify in 5 to 10 min). The capacity of the balloon necessary to occlude the fistula is now accurately measured and the balloon is totally deflated, but there is still iodine contrast material in both lumens of the catheter. The silicone-filled syringe is tightly adapted to one path of the catheter, directly, without any stopcock, which would add its own dead space and complicate the measurement of the proper amount of silicone to be injected. 0.3 ml of silicone is injected, corresponding to the dead space of each lumen of the catheter. One sees the balloon which is filled again with iodine contrast material. At that time, injection of silicone is momentarily stopped, and a 1-ml syringe attached to the second lumen of the catheter aspirates this 0.3 ml of iodine. The second lumen of the catheter is now tightly closed. Injection of silicone is resumed and the exact amount injected. An injection of contrast checks that the fistula is occluded without any leak of contrast in the cavernous sinus. The balloon is not radiopaque and only the silver tip is visible in the cavernous sinus. If the occlusion of the fistula is total, the first lumen of the catheter is also firmly closed. After the catalyzed silicone has solidified in the cup, the balloon can be detached. The double-lumen catheter is simply pulled out and if detachment is successful, the piece of silver will not move. An angiogram demonstrates the quality of occlusion of the fistula. The slightest mistake during replacement of iodine with silicone can mean that the balloon is not totally filled with silicone and will change its volume slightly after detachment. This causes a small leak of contrast around the balloon on the check angiogram. A small difference of inflation of 0.01 or 0.02 ml is enough to cause some leak. This leak will spontaneously disappear, or will increase, and it may be necessary to use a second balloon several days later, or the balloon, having become smaller, will be dislodged and will move within the cavernous sinus. In such a case, a second balloon will also be necessary.

Detachable Silastic balloons are also available (Becton–Dickinson, Heyer-Schulte). They have the advantage of being sterile and ready for use whenever needed. On the contrary, their lack of elasticity explains that a relatively small Silastic balloon, containing only 1 cc, will have to pass through a big introducer of 9F.

RESULTS OF BALLOON TREATMENT

Fifty-two patients with traumatic carotid cavernous sinus fistulas have been treated. All lesions were closed except one which was apparently closed after receiving one small balloon (0.1 ml) filled with iodine. An angiogram done 1 month later showed recurrence of this fistula because of two tiny branches of the siphon torn in the cavernous sinus. This patient is still asymptomatic and does not require a new balloon at present. The carotid blood flow was preserved in 60% of this series of patients. The internal carotid artery was occluded in the others because it was impossible to enter the cavernous sinus, or because of secondary thrombosis of the carotid siphon from the balloon bulging through the neck of the fistula, or because of a traumatic cervical dissection of the internal carotid artery at the time of the injury, or because of prior carotid artery ligation.

The complications were mainly oculomotor nerve palsies, retro-orbital pain, and false aneurysm. The oculomotor nerve palsies were frequent (20% of cases), the sixth nerve was more often involved than the third nerve. They happened more often when more than one balloon had to be detached in the cavernous sinus. The patients generally recovered after a few months. Permanent occlusion of the carotid artery may be necessary if oculomotor palsies are associated with a false aneurysm.

Pain from compression of the fifth nerve was generally transient. When it is a main symptom before treatment, it often instantaneously disappears as the fistula is occluded. It may be a problem after treatment when many balloons have been detached in the cavernous sinus. In one patient an inflammatory and edematous reaction of the eye occurred 2 weeks after occlusion of the fistula. Proptosis, chemosis, and edema of the lids suggested an active fistula, and the first impression was that the fistula had reopened despite the absence of a bruit. Angiogram demonstrated the absence of a fistula and a good carotid flow. All symptoms disappeared after several weeks with a good final result. Probably a secondary extensive thrombosis of the cavernous sinus explains this clinical course.

A false venous pseudoaneurysm occurred in 50% of the patients (Fig. 10A). Experience has shown that this pouch did not increase in size when it was small, did not cause TIAs, and afterwards spontaneously diminished in size (Fig. 10B). At times such a pouch is larger than 1 cm. If it increases in size on angiograms done at 6-month intervals, retreatment is proposed, with detachment of a second balloon inflated with silicone. If it is impossible to enter the pouch, permanent carotid occlusion has to be considered, or postponed if the patient is asymptomatic. It must be done if the patient is symptomatic (persistent pain or oculomotor nerve palsy). The use of double-lumen catheters is very recent but will probably avoid this inconvenience in the future or allow total occlusion of the venous pouch if needed.

EMBOLIZATION OF THE CAVERNOUS SINUS WITH BUCRYLATE THROUGH A CALIBRATED-LEAK BALLOON

This balloon has a small leak at the tip which opens when the balloon is fully inflated (Figs. 12 and 13). When it is in the cavernous sinus, bucrylate is injected through the balloon and solidified in the cavernous sinus. As soon as the bucrylate is injected, the balloon must be quickly removed to keep it from adhering to the cavernous sinus. This technique was used by Kerber (6) in a few cases of traumatic carotid cavernous fistulas. It should probably be reserved for cases which cannot be treated with a detachable balloon without occluding the carotid artery. With this technique come risks:

a) When the flow is fast and the cavernous sinus is wide, one cannot expect a complete thrombosis of the cavernous sinus. The quantity of bucrylate necessary to get this result would be more than can be safely used.

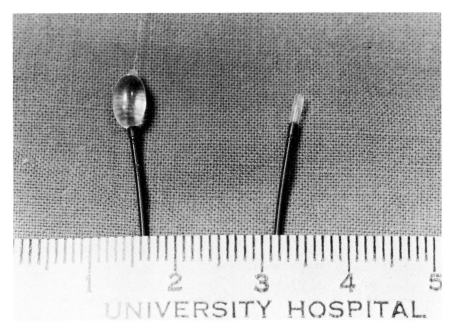

FIG. 12. Kerber calibrated leak balloon. Silastic balloon is attached to the tip of the Silastic tubing. The balloon has a distal calibrated leak. It cannot be detached.

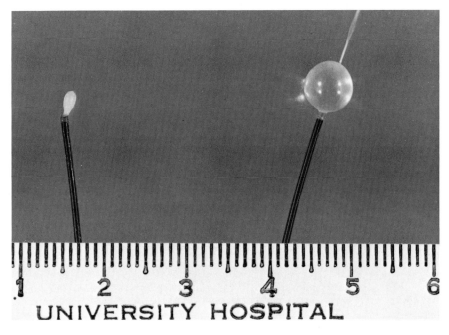

FIG. 13. Debrun calibrated leak balloon. Latex balloon grips the tip of the Silastic tubing without being attached; calibrated leak; the balloon can be detached by pulling the tubing.

b) An unknown quantity of bucrylate passes through the veins of drainage and embolizes the lungs. When the sinus is wide, almost all the injected bucrylate returns in solidified form to the lungs.

c) There is a risk of having some bucrylate escape from the cavernous sinus through the neck of the fistula and embolizing the internal carotid. Bucrylate injection should always be done with transient occlusion of the internal carotid artery below the fistula.

d) When bucrylate has been injected and the balloon catheter is quickly withdrawn there is again some risk of detaching some particles of bucrylate in the internal carotid artery.

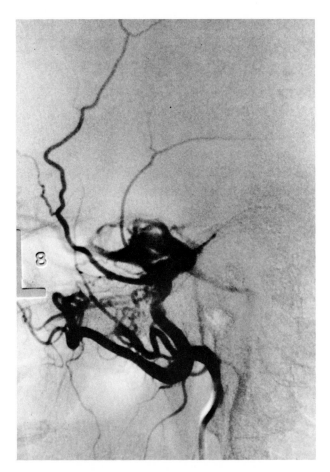

FIG. 14. Spontaneous dural AVM of the left cavernous sinus with a fistula. **A.** Meningeal branches from the external carotid.

e) Embolization of the cavernous sinus with bucrylate may induce an inflammatory reaction with pain lasting days or weeks.

f) This technique should be reserved for slow-flow fistulas with a small cavernous sinus, with almost intact partitions so that the quantity of bucrylate needed to occlude the neck of the fistula would be minimal.

TREATMENT OF SPONTANEOUS CAROTID CAVERNOUS SINUS FISTULA

Treatment differs from that of traumatic fistulas: a) It is impossible to enter the cavernous sinus with a balloon through the artery. b) Branches of the external carotid artery have to be embolized.

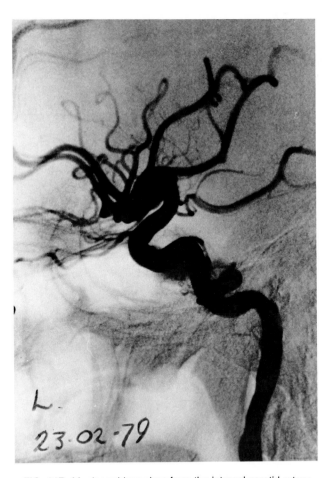

FIG. 14B. Meningeal branches from the internal carotid artery.

One should be less aggressive with this type of fistula than with traumatic cases, since some heal spontaneously. It would be a mistake to occlude the carotid siphon initially, because: a) The fistula would continue to be fed by external carotid branches. b) Many patients are cured by embolization of the external carotid branches only. c) These fistulas are often bilateral and treatment of the contralateral fistula would become more difficult and risky. d) It is always dangerous in an older patient to occlude a carotid siphon permanently.

The first step of treatment, when needed, is embolization of the meningeal branches of the external carotid artery. Embolization should be as selective as possible.

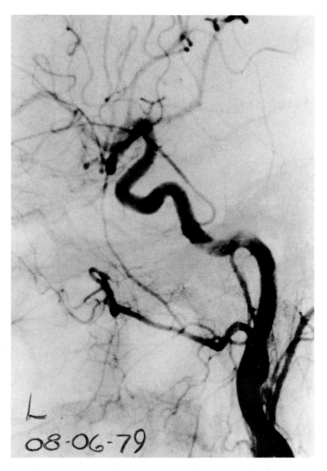

FIG. 14C. Angiography 4 months after embolization of the left internal maxillary artery with 0.5 ml of bucrylate. The fistula has gone, and the external carotid has recanalized. The internal carotid is normal, and the patient is asymptomatic.

The material used for embolization may be particles of Gelfoam, Ivalon or bucrylate. An example of dural AVM of the cavernous sinus with a fistula is shown in Fig. 14. Bucrylate (0.5 ml) was injected into the internal maxillary artery and reached the cavernous sinus, which thrombosed secondarily but with a painful inflammatory reaction and transient sixth nerve palsy. All the tiny branches between the carotid siphon and the cavernous sinus were occluded and the varix of the cavernous sinus which communicated with the siphon thrombosed.

Even after embolization with solid particles occluding the meningeal branches of the external carotid artery, spontaneous cure of the fistula often occurs, probably by spontaneous thrombosis of the cavernous sinus.

When embolization of the external carotid artery is not technically realized because of stenosis of the origin of the external carotid or of the bifurcation of the

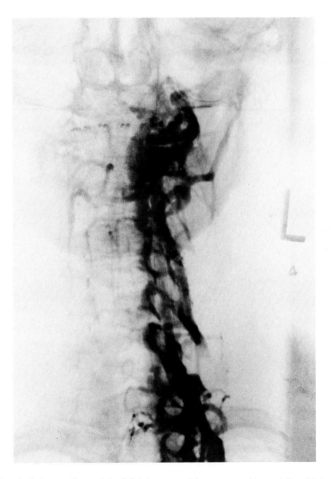

FIG. 15A. Left traumatic vertebral fistula caused by a screwdriver at the C6 to C7 level.

common carotid artery in an older patient, direct surgical approach of the cavernous sinus can be considered. Thrombosis can be obtained by injection of thrombogenic material (needles or wire) or particles such as pieces of Gelfoam, cotton, or pieces of muscle.

VERTEBRAL FISTULAS (Fig. 15)

Vertebral fistulas are also uncommon. They may be congenital or traumatic including iatrogenic fistulas after direct puncture of the vertebral artery. Iatrogenic fistulas are low in the neck, at C4 or C5 level. The congenital ones are at C1 to C2 level. It is difficult to say that true congenital fistulas exist, because a relatively mild injury can cause a fistula, as in one of our cases (the patient was hurt on the right side of the neck by the stick of a parasol when he was at the seashore). Mild

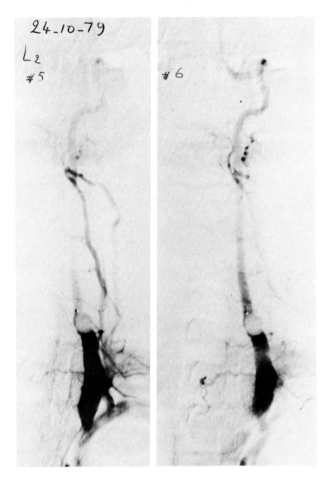

FIG. 15B. The balloon occludes the fistula but bulges into the vertebral artery which is almost completely occluded. The vertebral artery is still filled above the fistula through cervical arteries.

injury many years before discovery of the fistula may be forgotten by the patient. Obstetrical injury may cause such a fistula.

The anatomical particularity of fistulas at C1 to C2 is that their neck is generally very wide, necessitating a bigger introducer and bigger balloon than those used to treat a carotid cavernous fistula. There is also an almost constant participation of the ascending cervical arteries and of the occipital artery, which may either converge to the neck of the fistula or independently join the venous plexus of drainage. In the first case the occlusion of the fistula with one balloon will also occlude the connection with the ascending cervical artery and the occipital artery. The balloon may even be introduced through the occipital artery. In the second case, the occlusion of the neck of the fistula only closes the communication between the vertebral artery and the venous drainage plexus. The occipital artery and the ascending cervical artery have to be embolized separately. As the occipital artery may be widely communicating with the vertebral artery, and as the ascending cervical artery

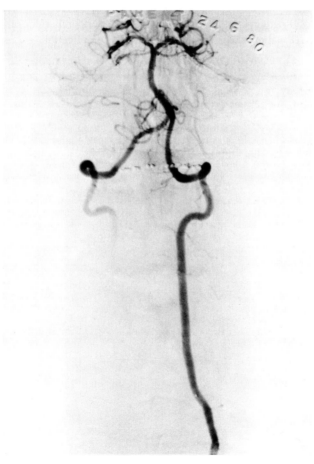

FIG. 15C. Six months after treatment the vertebral artery is normal.

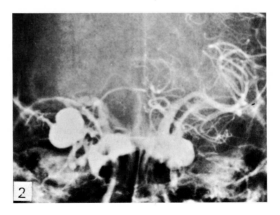

FIG. 2. (Same patient). Left-sided carotid angiogram (AP view). Note fistula on the left with drainage to the right ophthalmic vein.

fistula, especially as far as the sixth nerve is concerned. Vision loss present in two cases healed very quickly.

In all but two cases the fistula was closed by the balloon. In patient 4, it reopened first and closed spontaneously 48 hr later during an attempt to pass a new balloon into the fistula. Patient 11 gave problems due to rupture of the balloon, most probably resulting in enormous widening of the fistula with rapidly developing exophthalmus and deterioration of vision. An emergency Hamby procedure closed the fistula and restored his vision. We accepted the definite closure of the internal carotid. Non-deliberate closure of the carotid occurred spontaneously in patient 9 after the introduction of four balloons necessary to obstruct the huge fistula.

TABLE 1. *Nerve function before and after balloon occlusion*

Patient No.	Age and gender	Preexisting impaired nerve function	Nerve function 1 month post closure	Nerve function 1 yr post closure
1	58 F	N III and VI	Unchanged	Unchanged
2	22 M	N III and VI	N VI unchanged N III healed	N VI unchanged
3	54 F	Not impaired	Not impaired	Not impaired
4	30 M	N VII and VIII	N VII and VIII Unchanged	N VII and VIII Unchanged
5	29 M	Comatose	Comatose	
6	47 F	Not impaired	Not impaired	Not impaired
7	16 M	Not impaired	Not impaired	
8	28 M	N VII R + L	N VII R + L	
9	30 M	N III, IV and VI Vision 1/10	N III, IV and VI Improved Vision 10/10	
10	76 F	N VI Vision 1/60	N VI unchanged Vision 10/10	
11	25 M	Not impaired		
12	42 F	Not impaired		

TABLE 2. *Results of balloon occlusion*

Patient No.	Duration of procedure (hr)	No. of balloons	Volume (ml) in balloon	Results Immediately	1 month	1 year
1	4	1	0.5 silicone 0.1 contrast	Fistula closed	Fistula closed: pseudoaneurysm	Fistula closed; pseudoaneurysm
2	4	2	0.4 contrast 0.6 silicone 0.1 contrast	Fistula closed	Fistula closed: large pseudoaneurysm	Fistula closed; large pseudoaneurysm
3	3	1	0.5 silicone 0.1 contrast	Fistula closed: Carotid stenosis	Fistula closed: carotid stenosis disappeared	Fistula closed
4	3.5	1	0.8 silicone 0.1 contrast	Fistula opened after 48 hr Fistula closed spontaneously	Fistula closed	
5	2	—	—			Fistula closed
6	3	1	0.6 silicone 0.1 contrast	Fistula closed: carotid stenosis	Fistula closed: carotid stenosis	
7	6	2	0.5 silicone 0.1 contrast 0.6 silicone 0.1 contrast	Fistula closed	Fistula closed	Fistula closed
8	3	1	0.4 silicone 0.1 contrast	Fistula closed	Fistula closed	
9	4	4	0.6 silicone 0.6 silicone 0.7 silicone 0.5 silicone	Fistula closed: carotid closed	Fistula closed: carotid closed	Fistula closed carotid closed
10	3	1	0.1 silicone 0.1 contrast	Fistula closed	Fistula closed: pseudoaneurysm	
11	3	1	0.2 silicone 0.1 contrast	Fistula closed	Fistula closed	
12	4	—	—	Fistula not closed: balloons ruptured; Hamby procedure		
13	2	1	0.2 silicone 0.1 contrast	Fistula closed		

DISCUSSION

In the treatment of these 12 patients we encountered the following problems: (a) development of a pseudoaneurysm; (b) stenosis or complete occlusion of the carotid artery; (c) rupture of the balloon.

Development of a Pseudoaneurysm

During the exchange procedure of contrast medium against silicone, 0.1 ml of contrast medium representing the dead space of the catheter and deflated balloon remains in the balloon after filling with silicone. In the course of several weeks the contrast medium disappears due to diffusion through the wall of the balloon, thus diminishing the final content of the balloon by 0.1 ml (Fig. 3). Although the fistula remains closed, a pseudoaneurysm resulted at the site of the opening in the

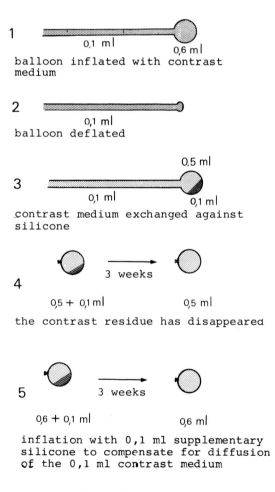

FIG. 3.   Balloon technique.

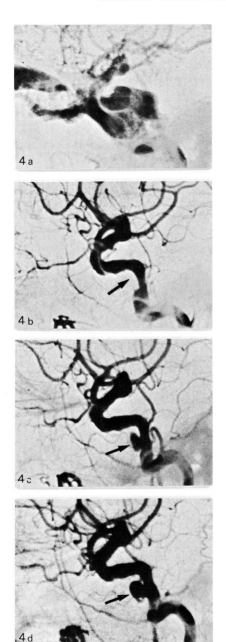

FIG. 4. (Patient 1). **a:** Lateral carotid angiogram shows cavernous sinus fistula prior to treatment. **b:** Appearance immediately after closure of the fistula with the aid of a balloon containing 0.5 ml of silicone and 0.1 ml of contrast medium *(arrow)*. **c:** One month after closure of the fistula, a small pseudoaneurysm *(arrow)* has developed due to diffusion of the residue of contrast medium.**d:** A year after closure of the fistula the pseudoaneurysm is unchanged *(arrow)*.

carotid artery (Fig. 4). In another case where we needed two balloons in order to obtain full closure of the fistula, one balloon was filled with contrast and the second one with silicone, as advocated by Debrun, to prevent compression of oculomotor nerves in the cavernous sinus. This procedure resulted in a large and even enlarging pseudoaneurysm after disappearance of the contrast medium (Fig. 5).

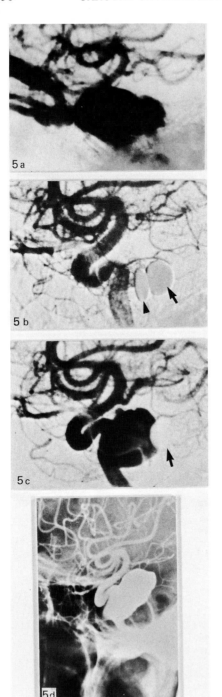

FIG. 5. (Patient 2). **a:** Lateral carotid angiogram shows cavernous sinus fistula prior to treatment. **b:** Appearance immediately after closure of the fistula with the aid of two balloons containing 0.4 ml of contrast medium *(arrow)* and 0.6 ml of silicone with 0.1 ml of contrast medium residue *(arrowhead)*. **c:** One month after closure of the fistula, the contrast medium in the second balloon has diffused and that in the first balloon has partly diffused *(arrow)*, causing a pseudoaneurysm. **d:** Two years after closure of the fistula the pseudoaneurysm remains unchanged.

Stenosis and Occlusion of the Internal Carotid

Since we have used an excess amount of 0.1 ml silicone during the exchange procedure, we have no longer observed the formation of pseudoaneurysms, but we have now seen transitory (Fig. 6) and, in one instance, permanent stenosis of the carotid artery without any clinical symptoms thus far.

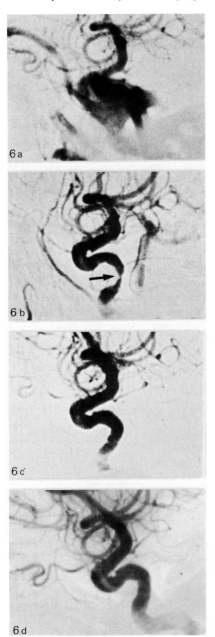

FIG. 6. (Patient 3). **a:** Lateral carotid angiogram shows cavernous sinus fistula prior to treatment. **b:** Appearance immediately after closure of the fistula with the aid of a balloon containing 0.5 ml of silicone and 0.1 ml of contrast medium. There is carotid stenosis *(arrow)* due to injection of a surplus of 0.1 ml silicone. **c:** One month after closure of the fistula, the carotid stenosis has been abolished as a result of diffusion of the residue of contrast medium. **d:** Appearance 1 year after closure of the fistula.

Complete occlusion of the carotid artery, fortunately without any consequences, has already been mentioned in patient 9 in whom the carotid became completely occluded during the introduction of four balloons and filling with silicone. The second case of complete occlusion of the carotid was patient 11 in whom a Hamby procedure performed as an emergency operation meant *ipso facto* interruption of the flow in the internal carotid.

Rupture of the Balloon

All balloons were manufactured by Ingenor, Paris, France. Rupture of one or more balloons occurred in 4 patients. In 3 patients silicone, still liquid, entered the circulation without giving rise to symptoms. In the fourth patient the rupture resulted probably in enormous widening of the fistula with rapidly progressing exophthalmos, papilledema, and deteriorating vision (patient 11). This patient is interesting in more than one respect. He is a 25-year-old man with a classical post-traumatic carotid cavernous fistula with exophthalmus, moderate oculomotor palsy, and a bruit over the left orbit. At the first attempt several balloons failed to enter the fistula. We decided to wait 4 weeks with close control of vision, fundus, and bruit, hoping for spontaneous enlargement of the fistula opening. This in fact happened, and, after 4 weeks, the bruit had become much louder and a second attempt was made. This time the balloon entered the fistula very easily, but, after filling with silicone well beneath capacity, the balloon ruptured. The top of the balloon came off at the moment of pulling at the catheter, entered the cerebral circulation and blocked one of the smaller branches of the gyri angularis artery, fortunately without any clinical symptoms (Fig. 7, **a, b,** and **c**).

Closure of the fistula in our series required from one to four balloons with a total volume of 0.2 to 2.4 ml. We prefer latex to silicone rubber as balloon material because of its greater elasticity. An empty latex balloon with a capacity of 0.6 ml measures 5×1.3 mm; when filled to capacity its dimensions are 18 mm in length and 8 mm in width. An empty silicone rubber balloon, however, with an equal capacity of 0.6 ml measures 7×1 mm; fully filled it measures only 16×4 mm. In our experience, rupture is more likely to occur when the balloon is introduced in a slender fistula than when it can expand symmetrically. In a slender fistula it may even occur before filling to capacity.

SUMMARY

Twelve patients with carotid cavernous fistulas treated with the detachable balloon technique are described. In 10, the fistula was closed by the balloon; 1 fistula closed spontaneously during balloon manipulation, and in 1 case no occlusion could be obtained, and balloon rupture led to complications necessitating a Hamby procedure. After a pseudoaneurysm had developed in the first 2 cases due to diffusion of contrast medium residue, slight silicone overfilling was used successfully in order to prevent this complication. However, this might have contributed to 1 permanent and 1 transient carotid stenosis and 1 case of carotid occlusion.

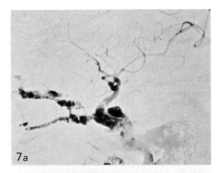

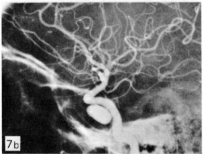

FIG. 7. (Patient 11). **a:** Lateral carotid angiogram shows cavernous sinus fistula prior to treatment. **b:** Appearance immediately after closure of the fistula with the aid of a 1 ml balloon containing 0.6 ml of contrast medium. **c:** After the exchange of the contrast medium against silicone, the balloon ruptured. The silver clip from the balloon moved to a branch of the middle cerebral artery *(arrow).* The procedure was interrupted.

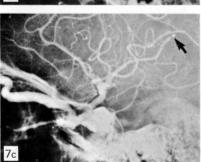

Although complications may occur, the detachable balloon technique is recommended provided it is used with the utmost care.

REFERENCES

1. Debrun, G., Lacour, P., and Caron, J. P. (1977): Balloon arterial catheter techniques in the treatment of arterial intracranial diseases. In: *Advances and Technical Standards in Neurosurgery* Vol. 4, edited by H. Krayenbuhl, pp. 131–145. Springer, New York.
2. Debrun, G., Lacour, P., Caron, J. P., Hurth, M., Comoy, J., and Kerevel, Y. (1978): Detachable balloon and calibrated-leak balloon techniques in the treatment of cerebral vascular lesions. *J. Neurosurg.*, 49:635–649.
3. Peeters, F. L. M., and van der Werf, A. J. M. (1980): Detachable balloon technique in the treatment of direct carotid-cavernous fistulas. *Surg. Neurol.*, 14:11.
4. Debrun, G., Lacour, P., Vimiela, F., Fox, A., Deake, Ch.G., Caron, J.P. (1981): Treatment of 54 traumatic carotid-cavernous fistulas. *J. Neurosurg.*, 55:678–692.

Vascular Malformations, edited by
R. R. Smith, A. Haerer and W. F. Russell.
Raven Press, New York © 1982.

Detachable Balloon Closure of Carotid Cavernous Fistula

*Thomas A. Tomsick, **John M. Tew, Jr., *Robert R. Lukin
and *Frank M. Eggers

*Departments of *Radiology and **Neurosurgery, Cincinnati General Hospital
and Good Samaritan Hospital, Cincinnati, Ohio 45267 and 45220*

Treatment of carotid cavernous fistulas leaving the internal carotid artery patent is now possible by percutaneous balloon techniques (2,3). Although we have achieved cure of fistulas in each of five attempts, each case presented a different problem in management. Our experiences are briefly detailed.

Case 1: A 20-year-old male developed chemosis, proptosis, and an orbital bruit several weeks after a motor vehicle accident. Internal carotid artery (ICA) angiography demonstrated a large carotid cavernous fistula (Fig. 1A). Puncture of the left common carotid artery was performed and three No. 17 Debrun detachable (Ingenor Medical, Paris, France) balloons filled with Conray 60 (Mallincrodt Pharmaceuticals) were detached within the fistula, but the fistula remained patent. As a fourth balloon was inflated to maximal filling volume (0.8 cc), the fistula closed completely, but the balloon ruptured. A fifth balloon was inflated to 0.75 cc and detached (Fig. 1B). The patient's proptosis and bruit diminished, but no more balloons were available. An immediate postembolization angiogram showed marked reduction in the flow of the fistula. Over the next 24 hr, the patient's bruit and exophthalmos disappeared. Angiography 7 days post-treatment confirmed closure of the fistula and patency of the internal carotid artery (Fig. 1C).

Note: Initial incomplete closure of the fistula may cause enough reduction of flow for subsequent total thrombosis.

Case 2: An 18-year-old male developed left proptosis and a bruit several months following an auto accident in which he suffered a basal skull fracture. A left ICA angiogram disclosed total flow into a large fistula (Fig. 2A). The left common carotid artery was cannulated. A prominent kink of the cervical internal carotid artery caused difficulty in passing the coaxial catheter system. The smaller Teflon catheter with balloon attached could be passed around the kink, but the combination of inner and outer catheters could not. A No. 17 balloon filled with 0.75 cc Conray 60 near completely occluded the fistula and was detached by pulling on the catheter system. The patient's symptoms and signs initially diminished, only to exacerbate in the following weeks.

Nine weeks later, the ICA was surgically exposed and a No. 17 Debrun balloon was easily passed into the fistula, and inflated, with complete fistula occlusion. The

241

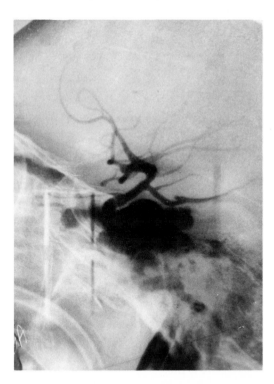

FIG. 1A. Lateral subtraction left ICA angiogram. High-flow ICA cavernous sinus fistula with drainage into the superior ophthalmic vein anteriorly and inferior petrosal sinus posteriorly.

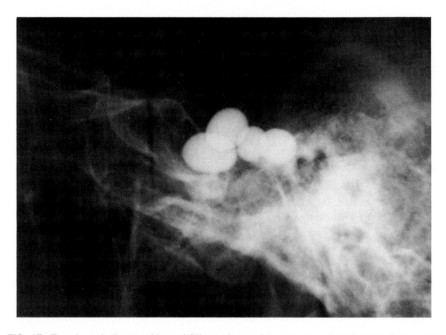

FIG. 1B. Four latex balloons with total filling volume of 2.6 cc were detached on the venous side of the fistula.

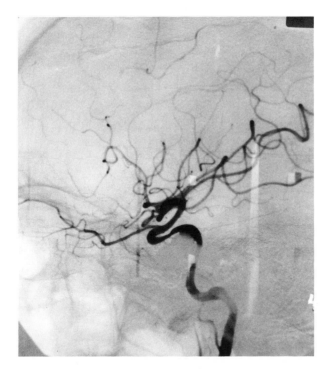

FIG. 1C. Post-treatment angiogram shows complete fistula closure and minimal narrowing of the cavernous ICA.

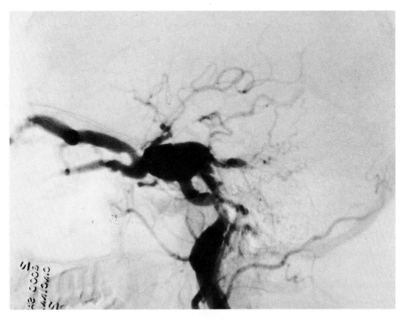

FIG. 2A. Lateral subtraction left ICA angiogram. ICA cavernous sinus fistula with drainage anteriorly into the superior and inferior ophthalmic veins and posteriorly into the superior and inferior petrosal sinuses and anterior pontomesencephalic vein.

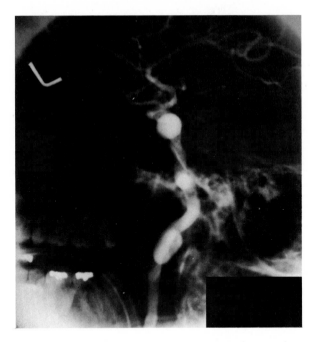

FIG. 2B. Detachment of one 0.75 cc contrast-filled balloon has occluded the fistula.

same difficulty was encountered with the ICA kink, and a pull-detachment was again performed (Fig. 2B). The patient remains symptom-free without bruit.

Note: Difficulty negotiating a kink in the ICA caused us to resort to balloon traction-detachment. Incomplete closure after the first treatment was not sufficient to initiate complete thrombosis.

Case 3: A 16-year-old male presented with slight proptosis, arterialization of the conjunctiva, and an orbital bruit 3 months after an auto accident in which he suffered a basal skull fracture. Angiography disclosed a large pseudoaneurysm of the internal carotid cavernous fistula (Fig. 3A). It appeared that percutaneous closure would be successful when inflation of a silicone balloon to 0.4 cc stopped flow into the fistula (Fig. 3B). However, on minimal further inflation, the balloon ruptured. Three more balloons ruptured in similar fashion.

Note: Repeated balloon rupture at approximately 50% maximum inflation volume was likely due to a fracture fragment or spicule at the fistula site.

A second elective closure was planned, but an episode of epistaxis (wherein the patient's blood pressure dropped to 70 systolic and his hematocrit fell 13 points) prompted definitive therapy.

Under direct surgical exposure, a larger Silastic balloon was passed into the fistula, but premature rupture again occurred.

One contrast-filled Silastic balloon and two latex balloons were then detached on the venous side of the fistula with near-complete closure. A fourth balloon would

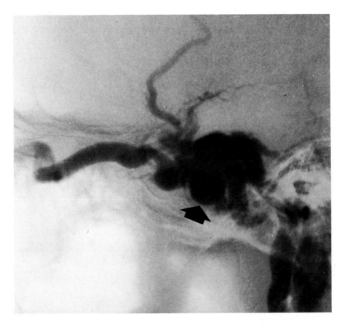

FIG. 3A. Subtracted lateral left ICA angiogram and cine angiography demonstrated a high-flow ICA cavernous sinus fistula with initial filling of the pseudoaneurysm *(closed arrow)*, and subsequent emptying into the cavernous sinus and connecting veins.

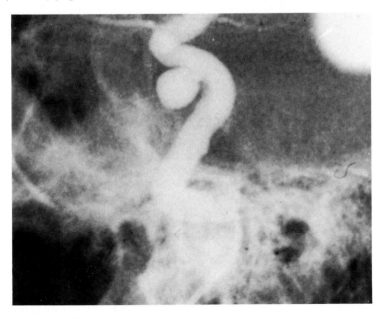

FIG. 3B. Closure of the fistula is shown prior to balloon detachment, but balloon rupture occurred subsequently.

not flow into the fistula, and was therefore detached in the juxtasellar ICA, and the ICA origin was ligated below. Signs and symptoms disappeared and postoperative angiography confirmed complete fistula closure.

Note: This patient's fistula had become life-threatening by virtue of erosion into the sphenoid sinus. Cure of the fistula and pseudoaneurysm was necessary. Due to the occurrence of pseudoaneurysms following fistula treatment with deflating water-soluble, contrast-filled latex balloons (2), near complete fistula closure was not acceptable in this case. Therefore, total ICA occlusion was chosen.

Case 4: A 38-year-old male suffered a gunshot wound to the face and orbit. Initially conscious in the emergency room, a right hemiparesis developed and the patient slowly lapsed into a coma. An orbital bruit was present. Plain films showed metallic fragments in the left orbit, zygomatic, and juxtasellar areas. Metallic artefact and patient motion on computerized tomography precluded diagnosis of a small pontine hemorrhage. Cerebral angiography demonstrated a left carotid cavernous fistula, and associated intimal damage of the cervical ICA (Fig. 4A).

Via the transfemoral route, a No. 17 Debrun latex balloon was passed into the fistula. Flow in the ICA seemed slower and more sluggish, and further spasm of the cervical ICA was evident. Balloon inflation to 0.4 cc maintained patency of the ICA with near complete fistula closure. Considerable traction was necessary to detach

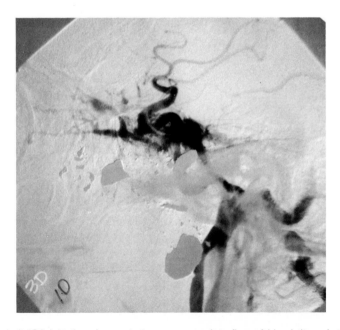

FIG. 4A. Left ICA injection demonstrates near complete flow of blood through the carotid cavernous fistula. Videotape indicated that the fistulous site was posterior and dorsal in location. Cervical ICA irregularity of minimal degree was likely due to simultaneous arterial damage by a bullet fragment. Cross filling from the right internal carotid artery to the fistula was present.

the balloon from the long transfemoral coaxial system. Serial films shortly after detachment showed slow flow in the internal carotid artery (Fig. 4B). Repeat angiography at 53 days showed left ICA occlusion and no filling of the fistula.

Note: Balloon detachment is more difficult with longer catheter systems via the transfemoral as opposed to the transcarotid route. Although this factor may have contributed to ICA occlusion, other damage to the ICA may have doomed this attempt from the inception.

Case 5: A 52-year-old woman complained of proptosis and swelling of her left eye, which was noted on arising one morning. There was no definite history of trauma. Physical examination demonstrated proptosis, a partial third nerve palsy, and prominent veins of the upper eyelid. A left temporal and supraorbital bruit was present. Cerebral angiography demonstrated a left carotid cavernous fistula, with near complete steal of blood to the fistula, and collateral flow into the left internal carotid artery distribution, through the anterior communicating arteries (Fig. 5A, and B).

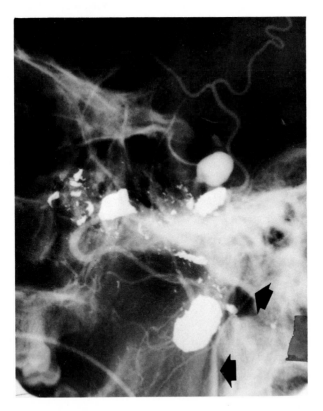

FIG. 4B. Lateral common carotid angiogram after balloon detachment. Filling of the external carotid artery branch is noted, with only a thin, dependent, layer of contrast seen in the internal carotid artery, with no flow past the inflated balloon *(arrows).*

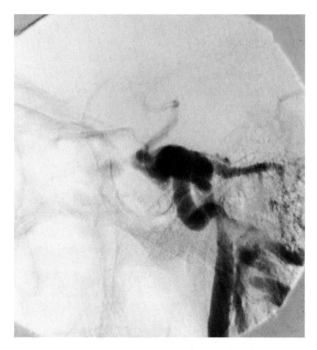

FIG. 5A. Lateral substrated internal carotid angiogram shows near complete flow of blood through the carotid cavernous fistula. Collateral flow to the internal carotid artery distribution through the posterior communicating arteries and anterior communicating arteries was also present.

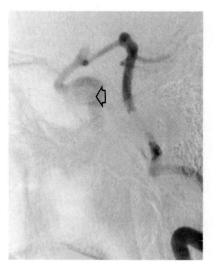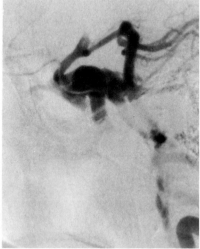

FIG. 5B. A subtracted, lateral vertebral artery angiogram with left common carotid compression indicates forward filling through the posterior communicating artery to internal carotid artery, down to the level of the fistula, judged to be at the junction of the presellar and juxtasellar segments of the internal carotid artery *(arrow)*.

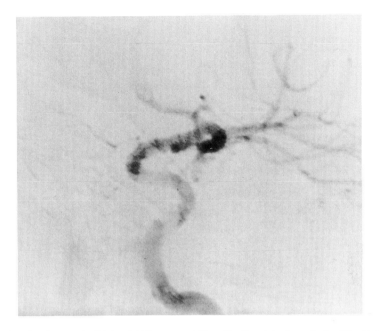

FIG. 5C. A subtracted off-lateral 105-mm spot film after the detachment of a Silastic balloon filled with 0.4 cc contrast material. Complete occlusion of the fistula is shown, with no flow through the cavernous sinus. The contrast filled balloon is subtracted from the angiogram.

Following cannulation of the common carotid artery, three 0.5 cc Silastic balloons were placed in the carotid cavernous fistula. All ruptured at various filling volumes from 0.35 to 0.5 cc. A fourth Silastic balloon totally occluded the fistula when inflated to 0.4 cc (Fig. 5C).

Note: Again, balloon rupture occurred prematurely, prior to inflation of the balloon to maximal filling volume. There was no evidence of basal skull fracture in this particular patient, and the nature of the premature rupture is still undetermined.

DISCUSSION

Each instance of carotid cavernous fistula presents a unique situation. Although closure of the fistula with patency of the ICA is the goal, this cannot be achieved in every case. Versatility in the use of balloon catheters, both detachable and nondetachable, and in the use of tissue adhesive expands the capabilities of the physicians managing this challenging therapeutic problem (1).

ACKNOWLEDGMENT

The authors wish to thank Drs. Lowell Ford, Phillip Minella, James McLennan, Thomas Berger, James Nichols, and George Prioleau for referring their patients for treatment.

REFERENCES

1. Berenstein, A., Kricheff, I. I., and Ransohoff, J. (1980): Carotid-cavernous fistulas: Intraarterial treatment. *AJNR*, 1:449–457.
2. Debrun, G., Lacour, P., Caron, J. P., Hurth, M., Comoy, J., and Keravel, Y. (1978): Detachable balloon and calibrated leak balloon technique in the treatment of cerebral vascular lesions. *J. Neurosurg.*, 49:635–649.
3. Peeters, F. L. M., and van der Werf, A. J. M. (1980): Detachable balloon technique in the treatment of direct carotid-cavernous fistulas. *Surg. Neurol.*, 14:11–19.

Subject Index

A

Acrylic embolization
  intracerebral hemorrhage during, 138
  intraoperative procedure for, 131–132
  and postembolization resection
    results in patients treated with, 133–135
  preoperative procedure for, 131
Air studies, in identification of AVMs, 33
Angioglioma
  classification of
    Bergstrand's, 14
    to differentiate between AVM and
      neoplasm, 14
Angiogram
  of dural AVM
    following embolization, 126
    showing arterial blood supply, 122
  following embolization
    for occipital temporal AVM, 152, 153
    for parietotemporal AVM, 143, 144, 145,
      146, 148, 150
    for thalamic AVM, 159, 160
  of large AVMs
    postembolization films of, 120–121
    postoperative, 82, 84, 86, 89, 91, 92, 95
    showing arterial blood supply, 80, 81, 83,
      84, 85, 89, 92, 93, 94, 119
    showing drainage, 85, 87
    showing residual abnormal vessels, 89, 90
    showing surface presentation, 82
  left intracranial carotid, 56
  postsurgical resection of occipital temporal
    AVM preembolization, 140, 141
  of spinal cord
    showing AVM, 113
    showing recanalization of artery, 115
Angiograms, in patients with AVMs, 5
Angiography
  in diagnosis of cavernous hemangioma, 38,
    44
  in diagnosis of vascular malformations
    failure of, 37–38
  follow-up
    importance of, 147, 156
  four vessel, 78
  of intracranial AVMs fed by external carotid
    artery, 36, 37
Angioma arteriovenosum
  classification of
    Bergstrand's, 14

to differentiate between AVM and
  neoplasms, 14
Angioma cavernosum, description of, 14
Angioma racemosum
  classification of
    Bergstrand's, 14
  description of, 14
Angioma racemosum arteriale
  classification of
    Bergstrand's, 14
  description of, 14
Angiomatous malformations, small,
  destruction of, 58
Angioreticuloma
  classification of
    Bergstrand's, 14
    to differentiate between AVM and
      neoplasm, 14
  description of, 14
Arteriogram
  of AVM arterial supply, 102, 106, 109, 111
    following pellet embolization, 103, 104,
      107, 114
  of intraluminal defect, 104
Arteriovenous aneurysms, *see* Arteriovenous
  malformations
Arteriovenous malformations (AVMs); *see*
  also under specific malformation
  of the brain
    activity at time of onset of, 3, 4, 11
    associated disorders with, 3, 4
    classifications associated with, 31, 32
    development of, 1, 25
    duration of symptoms prior to treatment
      in, 6
    effects on arterial and venous channels,
      27, 32, 33
    family history in, 3, 4
    follow-up data in patients with, 8–10, 12
    gigantism in, 32
    incidence of, 1, 2–3, 10
    location of lesions in, 5, 11, 25
    major feeding vessels of, 5, 6
    mortality in, 8, 10
    natural history of, 1–12
    onset of first bleed in, 6, 7
    presenting signs of, 3, 4
    presenting symptoms of, 3, 10
    rebleeding in, 7, 8
    sexual ratio in, 1, 10